THE COMPLETE
HIGH BLOOD PRESSURE DIET
COOKBOOK

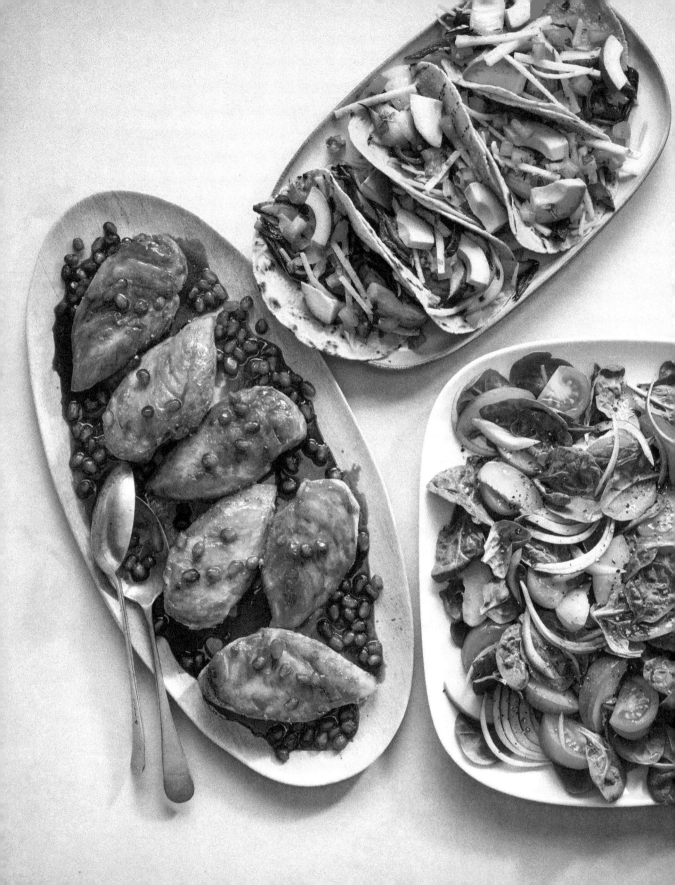

THE COMPLETE
HIGH BLOOD PRESSURE DIET
COOKBOOK

DASH Diet Recipes to Lower Blood Pressure and Improve Health

Edited by Amanda Foote, RD

Photography by Antonis Achilleos

ROCKRIDGE
PRESS

For my best friend, life partner, and loving husband, Alden

For general information on our other products and services or to obtain technical support, please contact our Customer Care Department within the United States at (866) 744-2665, or outside the United States at (510) 253-0500.

Rockridge Press publishes its books in a variety of electronic and print formats. Some content that appears in print may not be available in electronic books, and vice versa.

TRADEMARKS: Rockridge Press and the Rockridge Press logo are trademarks or registered trademarks of Callisto Media Inc. and/or its affiliates, in the United States and other countries, and may not be used without written permission. All other trademarks are the property of their respective owners. Rockridge Press is not associated with any product or vendor mentioned in this book.

Interior and Cover Designer: Carlos Esparza
Art Producer: Meg Baggott
Editor: Rachelle Cihonski
Production Editor: Sigi Nacson
Production Manager: Michael Kay

Photography © 2021 Antonis Achilleos
Food styling by Rishon Hanners
Author photo courtesy of Hardstep Designs

ISBN: 978-1-64876-326-7
eBook 978-1-64876-327-4

R0

Contents

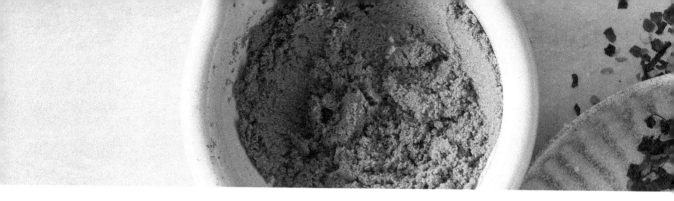

Introduction

Thank you for inviting me on your journey to blood pressure regulation using the power of nutrition. Being diagnosed with hypertension (high blood pressure) can be scary, but I assure you, you've come to the right place. Nutrition has been heavily studied and proven to be an effective tool in blood pressure management and reducing high blood pressure.

I am a registered dietitian, meaning my expertise is in how nutrition can be used therapeutically to heal the body. I am a food expert, and I am here to teach you how food can help you manage your high blood pressure. I have worked with people with hypertension for years—from adults with high blood pressure to specific populations like firefighters, who are more prone to developing high blood pressure—and I passionately believe that diet is an effective tool for blood pressure regulation.

This book will provide a comprehensive lifestyle and informational guide for those diagnosed with or interested in preventing high blood pressure, and includes 100 easy, healthy recipes to do so. The dietary approach discussed in this book is called the DASH diet (Dietary Approaches to Stop Hypertension). It is not an overly restrictive diet for rapid weight loss, nor is it a fad diet or elimination diet. Rather, it is a compilation of scientific dietary recommendations that are proven to reduce blood pressure. Every recipe in this book adheres to the DASH diet, and the recipes were carefully curated to ensure that you can enjoy healthier versions of your favorite dishes, not eliminate everything you love.

To get your taste buds excited, here are some recipes you can look forward to:

EGG SAUSAGE SANDWICH (page 43)—Yes, you can enjoy eggs and sausage (occasionally) on the DASH diet.

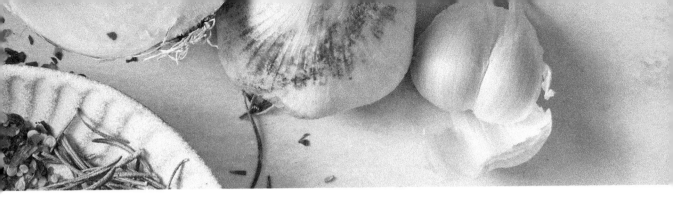

MAPLE-PECAN MASHED SWEET POTATOES (page 62)—Talk about sweet, savory, and creamy!

ROASTED VEGETABLE PIZZA (page 89)—More flavorful and satisfying than a greasy slice.

ARTICHOKE-STUFFED CHICKEN BREASTS (page 108)—Textures and flavors galore.

BUFFALO BURGERS (page 125)—Lean, flavorful, and delicious.

CHIPOTLE GUACAMOLE (page 143)—Even tastier when served with Baked Chili-Lime Tortilla Chips (page 140).

PEACH-BLUEBERRY CRISP WITH COCONUT TOPPING (page 152)—Satisfy that sweet tooth the healthy way.

Whether you've been recently diagnosed with high blood pressure or are simply looking for more healthy recipes to add to your repertoire and prevent hypertension, this book is a great resource for you. The DASH diet will very easily and quickly become the new way you eat, rather than a diet you "have to follow." You will find that food can taste even more flavorful with less salt and, instead, fresh ingredients, herbs, and spices. You will find that your favorites are just as good, or better, without the excess salt, fat, and added sugar. You will find that your groceries are no more expensive, your menu planning becomes streamlined, and you feel amazing from the nutrient-dense foods you are fueling your body with.

Welcome to *The Complete High Blood Pressure Diet Cookbook*.

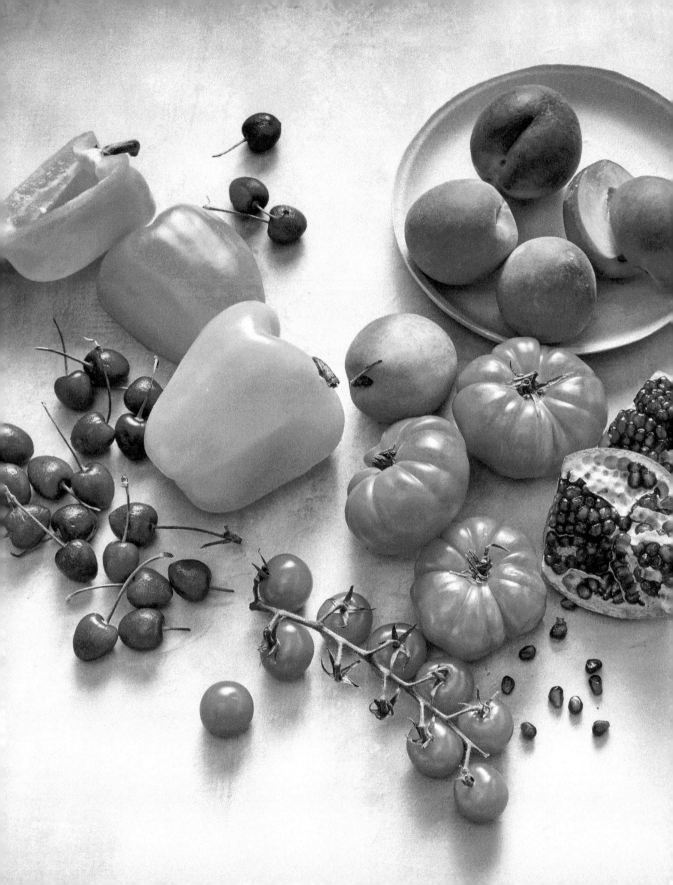

CHAPTER ONE

Living with and Reducing High Blood Pressure

Life with hypertension can be overwhelming. Getting the news from your doctor that your blood pressure is affecting your heart health can be scary, and people are often sent home with a new prescription but very little information on what they can do to improve their condition. My hope is that this book will be your comprehensive guide to managing, regulating, and lowering your blood pressure, and that it will instill confidence in you so you can take charge of your life and health with easy-to-apply dietary and lifestyle changes.

In this chapter, we will discuss what blood pressure is, the science behind high blood pressure, and what you can do to reduce your blood pressure with a few simple dietary, exercise, and lifestyle adjustments.

What Is High Blood Pressure and What Does It Mean?

Before we delve into what high blood pressure is, let's first talk about what blood pressure is. The action of the heart pumping pushes blood through the arteries (which carry blood from the heart out into the body). As the blood passes through the arteries, the blood puts pressure on the artery walls. It is normal for there to be pressure in the arteries from blood flow. It is also typical for blood pressure to fluctuate during the day and during different activities.

High blood pressure does not typically have noticeable symptoms until it has started to cause other health problems. It is a bit of a silent or invisible condition, which is why it is important to stay on top of your routine doctor's appointments to have your blood pressure checked regularly. Severe hypertension can cause symptoms like dizziness, vision changes, headaches, shortness of breath, or chest pain. If you experience any of these symptoms, you should seek medical attention immediately.

SYSTOLIC AND DIASTOLIC BLOOD PRESSURE

Systolic blood pressure is the top or first number in a blood pressure reading, and it indicates the amount of pressure in the arteries when your heart beats. Diastolic blood pressure is the bottom or second number in a blood pressure reading, and it indicates the amount of pressure in the arteries when your heart is resting in between beats.

A normal blood pressure measurement reads **120 SYSTOLIC** and **80 DIASTOLIC**, or **120 OVER 80**, or **120/80 MMHG**.

Elevated systolic blood pressure readings are usually the first risk factor for hypertension and heart disease; however, elevated diastolic blood pressure readings are also used for a high blood pressure diagnosis.

HOW IS HIGH BLOOD PRESSURE DIAGNOSED?

It is likely that your blood pressure is taken every time you visit a doctor (or the dentist) from childhood through adulthood. It is important that these readings are taken regularly to monitor your blood pressure trends to see if your pressure is stable, rising, or falling. Blood pressure is taken by a trained medical professional using a blood pressure cuff; your pressures are recorded and tracked by your health team.

If your blood pressure is elevated (between 120 and 129 systolic and less than 80 diastolic), your doctor may monitor your blood pressure more closely and recommend lifestyle changes to prevent you from developing hypertension.

Once your blood pressure reaches either 130 to 139 systolic or 80 to 89 diastolic, you may be diagnosed with stage 1 hypertension and your doctor likely will prescribe a blood pressure medicine as well as recommend lifestyle changes.

Once your blood pressure consistently reaches or exceeds 140 systolic and 90 diastolic, you may be diagnosed with stage 2 hypertension and your doctor will likely prescribe a combination of blood pressure medicines as well as recommend lifestyle changes.

If your blood pressure ever reaches or exceeds 180 systolic and 120 diastolic, you may be experiencing a hypertensive crisis, which requires immediate emergency medical attention.

PRIMARY AND SECONDARY HYPERTENSION

Most people diagnosed with high blood pressure have primary (also known as essential) hypertension. This kind of high blood pressure develops slowly over time and is caused by genetic predisposition, an increase in body weight, lack of exercise, lifestyle choices, and unhealthy dietary choices.

The other type of high blood pressure, secondary hypertension, has a more rapid onset and is caused by another medical condition such as sleep apnea, thyroid problems, kidney disease, or chronic substance use.

Blood Pressure by the Numbers

Reading	What it Means
Less than 120 systolic AND less than 80 diastolic	Normal blood pressure
120 to 129 systolic AND less than 80 diastolic	Prehypertension
130 to 139 systolic OR 80 to 89 diastolic	Stage 1 high blood pressure
140 or higher systolic OR 90 or higher diastolic	Stage 2 high blood pressure
180 or higher systolic AND/OR 120 or higher diastolic	Hypertensive crisis

RISK FACTORS FOR AND OUTCOMES OF HIGH BLOOD PRESSURE

In the United States, close to half of adults have high blood pressure over 130 systolic or 80 diastolic, and only about a quarter of that population has their blood pressure under control. About half of people with uncontrolled hypertension have stage 2 hypertension.

People who develop high blood pressure are more likely to regularly eat high-salt foods, drink excessive amounts of caffeine or alcohol, not exercise enough, smoke, and/or have poor sleep habits. High blood pressure puts you at greater risk for heart attack, stroke, heart disease, heart failure, kidney damage, vision problems, dementia, and premature death.

Demographics

Along with genetics and lifestyle, demographics also play a factor in who is most likely to develop high blood pressure. The age demographic with the highest incidence of high blood pressure is those age 60 and above, followed by adults ages 40 to 59; the lowest rates are seen in adults ages 18 to 39 years old. This makes sense, because as we age, our arteries naturally harden and lose their flexibility, which naturally causes an increase in blood pressure. Also, the longer unhealthy lifestyle choices have been going on, the longer they have had to negatively affect your health. Smoking for thirty years causes more damage than smoking for one year.

Men are more likely to develop hypertension than women, though women's risk does increase after menopause. This discrepancy is primarily because women are more likely to stay regular with their doctor's appointments than men, and are more likely to take preventative measures for their health than men.

Regarding ethnicity, Black people are the most likely to develop high blood pressure, followed by Caucasian people, Hispanic people, and then non-Hispanic Asian people. A large number of people with high blood pressure live in the southern United States and in low-income areas, where systemic societal differences have hastened the rise in blood pressure. These differences include food deserts where quality fresh, whole foods are not easily accessible, causing people to rely on high-fat/high-sodium convenience foods for nutrition; lack of access to quality insurance coverage; limited access to adequate health care; language barriers; and an inability to afford prescription medication.

DASH Diet and Lifestyle Changes to Lower High Blood Pressure

The best news is that blood pressure can often be reduced naturally with diet and exercise. We will be focusing heavily on diet in this book, but we will also discuss key lifestyle changes that you can implement immediately, with little to no stress.

DIET

Diet is the number one way to heal the body and prevent illness from the inside out. The nutrients in the foods you eat power every cell of your body. Feeding your body healthy foods is like giving your car oil and gas, but feeding your body processed foods and junk food is like depriving your car of oil and giving it the wrong kind of gas. We, like cars, are performance machines, and we need the right fuel to work properly.

This book is not meant to demonize any food. Sugar and fat are not inherently "evil"—they are just not your body's preferred sources of fuel. A diet consisting of processed foods, fast foods, and sugary, salty, oily, and fried foods is associated with excess weight gain; high blood pressure, cholesterol, and blood sugar; low energy; and increased fatigue. A diet focusing on more whole foods, such as fruits and vegetables, whole grains, and lean proteins, can help maintain a healthy weight, normal blood pressure and blood sugar, good cholesterol, and increased energy and stamina.

The DASH diet has been proven to be the best way to lower and control high blood pressure. It is also effective in preventing diabetes, heart disease, stroke, cancer, and osteoporosis. While this book specifically focuses on the DASH diet, there are other, similar eating patterns that also can help reduce blood pressure, such as the Mediterranean diet, as well as vegan, vegetarian, and pescatarian diets.

THE DASH DIET

Created by the National Heart, Lung, and Blood Institute (NHLBI), a branch of the National Institutes of Health (NIH), the DASH diet was intended to combat the high blood pressure epidemic in America. It is not a diet in the sense you might fear: It does not call for juice cleanses or fasting. Rather, it is a healthy eating plan that focuses on creating sustainable lifestyle changes that can help regulate blood pressure and improve heart health.

The diet emphasizes consuming easy-to-find, heart-healthy foods, rather than specialty, expensive so-called health foods. All you need to be successful on the DASH diet are a grocery store and some basic kitchen tools. The DASH diet also emphasizes proper portion sizes and healthful cooking methods. For example, zucchini is perfectly healthy, until you deep-fry it in oil and coat it with cheese. At its core, the DASH diet recommends eating:

- Beans and legumes (4 to 5 servings per week)
- Fruits (4 to 5 servings per day)
- Lean poultry and fish (6 ounces or less per day)
- Low-fat or fat-free dairy products (2 to 3 servings a day)

- Nuts and seeds (4 to 5 servings per week)
- Vegetables (4 to 5 servings a day)
- Vegetable oil for cooking (2 to 3 tablespoons a day)
- Whole grains (6 to 8 servings a day)

The diet also recommends limiting:

- Added salt (The goal is 1,500 to 2,300mg of sodium per day—the majority of recipes in this book are low in sodium to keep you on the lower end of this range and to allow sodium intake in other areas of your life, such as when you would like a sprinkle of salt at the table, a sports drink, or a meal out.)

- Added sugar, sweetened beverages, and baked goods (5 servings or less per week)
- Alcohol (maximum two drinks a day for men, one drink a day for women)
- Caffeine (in moderation, such as two 8-ounce cups or less of coffee per day)

- Saturated fats, including fatty meats and full-fat dairy, including butter (as limited as possible)

- Trans fats, including baked goods and fried foods (as limited as possible)

MAINTAINING A HEALTHY WEIGHT

Weight loss can help lower blood pressure. Excess weight is directly associated with the same diet and lifestyle choices that cause and worsen high blood pressure. Maintaining a healthy weight is a great way to combat high blood pressure because there is less stress on the body, and less stress on the heart and how hard it needs to pump. Excess body fat can cause insulin resistance, which increases sodium reabsorption; this, in turn, raises blood pressure and puts additional stress on the kidneys—which also raises blood pressure.

A good metaphor to think of would be if you have a pickup truck (your cardiovascular system), and are trying to use it to tow a full semi-trailer (excess body weight). Your truck's engine will be under a lot more stress than if you were only trying to tow a small travel trailer (healthy body weight). Keys to maintaining a healthy weight include eating a diet low in excess fat and added sugar and high in lean protein, vegetables, fruits, fiber, healthy fats, and whole grains.

REGULAR EXERCISE

Regular exercise is important for all people, and it is particularly beneficial for anyone with high blood pressure. Regular exercise is extremely good for the cardiovascular system, and while exercise temporarily elevates your blood pressure from activity, over time, it can lower your resting blood pressure. This is because exercise improves how well our body utilizes oxygen, creating less work for the heart to pump blood. It reduces stress hormones that harm the heart, increases good cholesterol, and lowers bad cholesterol.

The ideal exercise for the heart is a combination of aerobic exercise and resistance training—for example, biking and gentle weight lifting. The good news is that heart-healthy exercise takes countless forms, and you do not have to do anything you do not want to do. You do not have to run if you dislike running! Aerobic activity includes heavy housework like mowing the lawn or scrubbing floors, any sport you enjoy playing, walking, biking, swimming, and dancing. For resistance exercise like weight lifting, you can do body-weight exercises (no additional weight added), use resistance bands or weight machines at a gym, or try traditional weight lifting using barbells or hand weights.

Your exercise goal should be 150 minutes per week, which you can break down however you like. You could do five 30-minute sessions per week, or two 20-minute sessions per day—or whatever configuration best fits your lifestyle.

Different types of exercise that are easy on the body, easy to start doing, and require no special equipment or training include walking, yoga, exercise videos (free on the internet), body-weight exercises (free on the internet), and dance videos (free on the internet).

It can feel daunting to embark on an exercise plan along with a new diet, but the easy recipes in this book are meant to facilitate a lifestyle where there is more time for exercise. Instead of spending all night in the kitchen, you can squeeze in some exercise before you cook dinner. Use the following table as an example of what a gradual workup to a new exercise routine could look like.

Exercise	Week 1	Week 2	Week 3	Week 4
Walking	15 minutes every other day	20 minutes every other day	20 minutes every day	30 minutes 5 times per week

MEDICATION

Your doctor may have prescribed one or more medications for your high blood pressure. These medications are effective at controlling and lowering blood pressure to a healthy level. It is imperative that you take your medications as prescribed. High blood pressure medications fall into many different categories. You can use the following list as a general guide to these categories, but your doctor is the best resource for understanding your options.

DIURETICS: Remove excess salt and water from the body

BETA-BLOCKERS: Reduce heart rate and the heart's workload

ACE INHIBITORS: Relax narrowed blood vessels

ANGIOTENSIN II RECEPTOR BLOCKERS: Prevent blood vessels from constricting

CALCIUM CHANNEL BLOCKERS: Relax narrowed blood vessels and reduce heart rate

ALPHA-BLOCKERS: Reduce arterial resistance

ALPHA-2 RECEPTOR AGONISTS: Decrease adrenaline

COMBINED ALPHA- AND BETA-BLOCKERS: Reduce the heart's workload and arterial resistance

CENTRAL AGONISTS: Prevent blood vessels from tensing up

PERIPHERAL ADRENERGIC INHIBITORS: Reduce blood pressure by changing the neurotransmitters in the brain

VASODILATORS: Relax and widen blood vessels

OTHER LIFESTYLE CHANGES

Along with diet, exercise, and medication, there are several other lifestyle changes you can make to lower your blood pressure or prevent it from increasing.

QUIT SMOKING: Smoking is a proven hypertensive, which means it stimulates the sympathetic nervous system, raising blood pressure. Smoking also directly reduces the lungs' ability to use oxygen, which strains the heart, causes arterial stiffness, and creates inflammation. It is extremely important to quit smoking if you have high blood pressure.

LIMIT ALCOHOL CONSUMPTION: Similarly, drinking alcohol in quantities higher than the recommended limits causes temporary increases in blood pressure, but repeated drinking causes long-term elevations to blood pressure. Alcohol can also cause weight gain because it contains calories, and excess weight raises blood pressure.

REDUCE STRESS: Stress is also a common cause of elevated blood pressure. Stress releases stress hormones in the body, which damage your arteries. The great news is that regular exercise is proven to reduce stress. Exercises like yoga and meditation are effective at both reducing stress and lowering blood pressure.

Guidelines for Your DASH Kitchen

As we move into the practical application of the DASH diet, let's discuss the diet in a bit more depth. The important elements of the DASH diet are to eat plenty of foods that are low in fat and salt and high in vitamins, minerals, and antioxidants. That may sound limiting or overwhelming, but when you walk into the grocery store, nearly every whole food is DASH diet friendly.

You can enjoy every food in the fresh produce section; fresh or frozen lean cuts of meat and poultry from the meat department; fresh or frozen seafood; breads, pasta, rice, cereals, and grains from the dry goods aisles; dried fruits, seeds, and nuts; frozen fruits and vegetables from the frozen food section; and eggs and low-fat dairy from the dairy department. Really the only aisles you will be limiting your shopping in are the junk food aisles that contain chips, crackers, cookies, candy, soda, bakery desserts, and frozen desserts.

FOODS TO ENJOY

The foods that you are welcome to enjoy are effective at lowering your blood pressure due to being low in fat and salt and high in fiber, vitamins, and minerals. Bookmark this handy table for examples of each food category, how many servings to aim for each day, as well as why these foods are great for reducing hypertension.

A NOTE FOR USING THIS TABLE: Serving sizes do matter. A gigantic plate of whole-grain pasta is not one serving—it is likely 4 or 5 servings.

Food category	Examples	Recommended servings	Serving size examples	Why it's great for reducing high blood pressure
Whole Grains (amaranth, barley, buckwheat, bulgur, corn, farro, fonio, freekeh, millet, oats, quinoa, rice, rye, sorghum, teff, triticale, wheat, wild rice)	Bread, brown rice pilaf, hot cereal, tortilla chips, crackers, oatmeal, pasta, popcorn, cooked quinoa	6 to 8 per day	1 slice bread; 1 ounce dry cereal; ½ cup cooked cereal, rice, or pasta	Whole grains are high in fiber and heart-healthy vitamins and minerals like folate, iron, magnesium, potassium, and selenium. Whole grains keep you feeling full for longer, decrease insulin resistance, and reduce damage to the blood vessels.

Food category	Examples	Recommended servings	Serving size examples	Why it's great for reducing high blood pressure
Fruit (fresh, frozen, dried, or canned in 100% juice or light syrup)	Any fruit you like, including: apples, apricots, avocados, bananas, berries, cherries, figs, grapes, kiwifruits, lemons and limes, mangoes, melons, oranges, papayas, peaches, pears, pineapples, plums	4 to 5 per day	1 medium fruit; ¼ cup dried fruit; ½ cup cut fresh, frozen, or canned fruit	Fruit is full of vitamins, minerals, and antioxidants that are heart healthy and blood pressure reducing, and naturally low in sodium. Similar to whole grains, the fiber, potassium, and magnesium in fruits are blood pressure lowering.
Vegetables (fresh, frozen, or canned in water, no salt added or low sodium)	Any vegetable you like, including: asparagus, beets, broccoli, Brussels sprouts, cabbage, carrots, celery, cucumbers, eggplant, endives, green beans, kale, lettuce, mushrooms, peppers, potatoes, radishes, spinach, squash, sweet potatoes or yams, tomatoes, turnips, zucchini	4 to 5 per day	1 cup raw leafy greens; ½ cup cut raw or cooked vegetable	Vegetables are also low in sodium, high in fiber, and high in vitamins, minerals, and antioxidants that are heart healthy and blood pressure reducing. Leafy green vegetables in particular are high in nitrates, which are proven to reduce blood pressure.

continued →

Food category	Examples	Recommended servings	Serving size examples	Why it's great for reducing high blood pressure
Dairy (low-fat or fat-free)	Milk, cheese, cottage cheese, cream cheese, sour cream, yogurt	2 to 3 per day	8 fluid ounces low-fat milk; 1 cup plain low-fat yogurt; 1½ ounces low-fat cheese	Low-fat diets with high consumption of low-fat dairy are proven to lower systolic blood pressure by up to 3.5 points. Low-fat dairy is still high in potassium and magnesium.
Nuts, Seeds, and Legumes	Almonds, Brazil nuts, cashews, chestnuts, flaxseed, hazelnuts, macadamia nuts, nut butters, peanuts, pecans, pine nuts, pistachios, pumpkin seeds, sesame seeds and tahini, soybeans or soy nuts, sunflower seeds, walnuts; black beans, cannellini beans, chickpeas (garbanzo beans), great northern beans, lentils, lima beans, navy beans, peas	4 to 5 per week	⅓ cup whole nuts; 2 tablespoons nut butter; 2 tablespoons seeds; ½ cup cooked beans or peas	Nuts and seeds are great blood-pressure reducers due to their high levels of magnesium, heart-healthy fat, and fiber. Beans and legumes are also high in fiber and rich in vitamins and minerals important for heart health. Nuts and seeds are high in omega-3 fatty acids that reduce inflammation in the body, naturally decreasing blood pressure and improving heart health. Choose unsalted nuts and seeds and their butters, and low-sodium or no-salt-added canned beans and legumes.

Food category	Examples	Recommended servings	Serving size examples	Why it's great for reducing high blood pressure
Poultry, Fish, and Other Lean Meats	Beef sirloin, beef top round, beef flank steak, bison (buffalo), lamb, pork tenderloin or chops (fat trimmed), venison; chicken or turkey breast, (skinless); cod, crab, flounder, haddock, halibut, lobster, mackerel, pollock, salmon, sardines, shrimp, sole, squid and octopus, tilapia, trout, tuna; eggs and egg whites	Up to 6 ounces (cooked) per day	1 ounce cooked meat, poultry, or fish; 1 egg; 2 egg whites	Meat itself is not required for the DASH diet. If you do eat meat, the key is to choose lean cuts. Lean animal proteins are healthy in limited amounts, quantities much lower than the typical American is accustomed to eating. The DASH diet is much heavier on whole grains, fruits, vegetables, and plant-based proteins like beans, legumes, and nuts. Fish, on the other hand, are incredibly heart healthy due to their high omega-3 fatty acid content, a natural anti-inflammatory that decreases pressure and constriction in your blood vessels.

continued →

Food category	Examples	Recommended servings	Serving size examples	Why it's great for reducing high blood pressure
Healthy Fats and Oils	Avocado oil, canola oil, corn oil, nonstick cooking spray (avocado, canola, olive, or vegetable oil), olive oil, peanut oil, safflower oil, soybean oil, sunflower oil	2 to 3 per day	1 teaspoon oil; 2 tablespoons low-fat dressing	Similar to omega-rich fish, nuts, and seeds, you can get your inflammation-fighting omega fatty acids from the cooking oil you choose.

FOODS TO LIMIT

Though there are countless foods you can enjoy on the DASH diet, there are also some foods that you should limit. Remember, DASH is not an elimination diet, so you can still enjoy these foods *sometimes*. You don't have to say good-bye to the things you love; you just need to find ways to enjoy them in smaller portions, and less frequently. For example, instead of three scoops of ice cream after dinner every night, you can enjoy one scoop of ice cream twice a week and eat fresh fruit for dessert other nights throughout the week.

Red Meat

Red meat includes beef, lamb, pork, buffalo, venison, and others. The DASH diet recommends that red meat consumption be as limited as possible. For the purposes of this cookbook and the diet, "as limited as possible" will be the same as the lean protein recommendation of 6 ounces or less per day. Red meat should not be your choice daily, but keeping it in your weekly meal rotation is still healthy.

Sweets and Dessert

These treats fall into the category of added sugar, sweetened beverages, and baked goods. The goal on the DASH diet is to limit these foods to five servings or less per week. A serving size is considered 1 tablespoon of sugar or sweetener, 1 tablespoon of jam, ½ cup of sorbet, or an 8-fluid ounce serving of a sugar-sweetened beverage.

So, for instance, if you love sugar in your coffee, perhaps use 1 teaspoon of sugar per cup instead of 2 tablespoons. If baked goods are your weakness, enjoy one or two per week. If soda is your kryptonite, enjoy an 8-ounce glass a couple of times per week, or switch to sugar-free or diet soda (which should also be limited).

The dessert recipes in chapter 7 are healthy options, but should still be enjoyed with moderation in mind, meaning five or fewer servings per week.

Saturated and Trans Fats

These types of fat are the opposite of heart healthy, clogging and damaging your arteries instead of helping them stay clear and open. Saturated and trans fats should be as limited as possible on the DASH diet. Saturated fat is found in foods like butter, lard, coconut oil, cake, fatty cuts of meat, sausage, bacon, deli meats, regular-fat cheese and milk, pastries, ice cream, sour cream, and cream cheese.

Trans fats are often found in these same foods but are most commonly found in fried foods (fries, doughnuts, fried chicken, fast food), shortening, and freezer meals like frozen pizzas. Most of these foods are easy to avoid, but if you rely on deli meat for sandwiches, try to cook an extra chicken breast during the week and slice or shred it for your sandwiches, or choose tuna instead. Good alternatives to this category of foods are fat-free cheeses, low-fat milk, or homemade baked goods. I know that a lot of these foods are delicious, like a big greasy slice of pepperoni pizza (which you can indulge in on rare occasion), but try to remember the damage it is doing directly to your body and your blood pressure, and maybe it will be easier to say no thank you.

Sodium

Sodium, while not really a food group, gets a special mention because keeping track of it is so essential to managing your blood pressure. To help manage your blood pressure, added salt should be limited. Sodium is a naturally occurring element in our food and soil and is vital to survival, but in much smaller quantities than the average American is consuming. If you cut out all added salt, you will still be getting enough to stay healthy, don't worry!

The goal on the DASH diet is to limit total sodium intake to 1,500mg to 2,300mg per day. The majority of recipes in this book are under 500mg of sodium per serving to help you stay on the lower end of this range. This is also a great time to remind you that giving up added salt does not mean you have to sacrifice flavor. Herbs, spices, and acids are great for adding flavor when salt isn't an option. Purchasing no-salt-added or low-sodium products ensures that each serving has 5 percent or less of your daily recommended sodium.

You may have seen salt substitutes on the market, but this book uses none of them. Rather, we will rely on the natural flavor of the foods, seasoned with rich herbs and spices, proving to your palate that you do not need added salt (or fake salt) to enjoy amazing meals.

Hopefully, staying committed to the DASH diet, your taste buds will naturally come to enjoy herbs and spices, and you will likely find added salt to be abrasive and too strong for your palate. We have crafted the recipes in this book knowing that you may wish to add a pinch of salt to your food at the table if absolutely necessary for flavor, but always keep in mind that the goal is to stay under the max of 2,300mg of sodium a day. A pinch of salt here and there is better than giving up on the DASH diet entirely, but the hope is that you will ultimately learn to eat and cook without it.

Simple Swaps

There are tons of swaps you can try to make anything heart healthier and blood pressure–friendly, like cauliflower rice for white rice. These swaps are simple, inexpensive, and sensible. Not to mention they still taste great!

Instead of . . .	Try . . .
White rice	Brown rice, cauliflower rice, wild rice
Sour cream	Plain low-fat Greek yogurt
Butter on white toast	Drizzle of olive oil or slice of avocado on whole-wheat toast
White bread, bagels, or English muffins	Whole-grain bread, bagels, or English muffins
White pasta	Lentil pasta, veggie noodles, whole-grain pasta
Flavored, sweetened instant oatmeal from a packet	Steel-cut or old-fashioned oatmeal with fruit
Strawberry ice cream	Homemade fruit sorbet (just fruit and ice)
Mozzarella cheese on takeout pizza	Skim mozzarella cheese on homemade pizza

Instead of . . .	Try . . .
Cheddar cheese on beef tacos	Low-fat Cheddar cheese and extra veggies on turkey tacos
8-ounce porterhouse steak with loaded mashed potatoes	4-ounce sirloin steak with broccoli and wild rice
Any regular canned beans or vegetables	No-salt-added or low-sodium beans (if you cannot find them, drain the liquid from the can and rinse the beans well in a strainer to remove up to half the added salt)
Any regular canned fruit in heavy syrup	Choose fruits canned in 100 percent juice, light syrup, or no sugar added; you can drain the juice to reduce the sugar content
Ranch dressing on salad	Oil and vinegar on salad
Fried chicken thighs	Baked skinless chicken breast
Sandwich with mayonnaise and deli meat	Avocado and tuna sandwich

Healthy Kitchen Staples and Essentials

Success on the DASH diet starts in the kitchen. To prepare yourself for the lifestyle change, overhaul your pantry, fridge, and freezer by stocking up on some DASH-friendly powerhouses and reducing foods that are not heart healthy and will hinder your progress to achieving healthy blood pressure levels.

FOODS TO STOCK UP ON

Bookmark this section to make a list for stocking your pantry, fridge, and freezer with foods you should look for at the grocery store so that you always have the essentials to prepare DASH-friendly meals and snacks. Also, refer to the Foods to Enjoy chart on page 10 to help you build your list out further. Of course, you might need specific ingredients, or need to purchase fresh bread, produce, and meat items to make the recipes in this book, but these basics are essential to get you started on the right foot.

Pantry

- Broth or stock, low-sodium chicken or vegetable
- Brown rice (instant is fine)
- Canned beans (pinto, black, kidney, chickpeas, etc.), low-sodium or no-salt-added, if possible
- Canned fruit (peaches, pears, oranges, pineapple) in 100% juice, water, or light syrup, if possible
- Canned tomatoes, tomato sauce, tomato paste, no-salt-added
- Canned tuna, packed in water, no-salt-added
- Canned vegetables, low-sodium or no-salt-added, if possible
- Canola or corn oil
- Cereal (cornflakes, whole-grain square cereal, whole-grain toasted oat), unsweetened
- Dried beans (pinto, black, kidney, red) and lentils

- Dried fruit (raisins, prunes, apricots, bananas, strawberries), unsweetened
- Nonstick cooking spray (avocado, canola, olive, or vegetable oil)
- Nut butters, low-sodium or no-added-sugar
- Nuts and seeds of any kind, raw unsalted
- Oats, steel-cut or old-fashioned
- Oil (olive, avocado, canola, or vegetable)
- Popcorn kernels
- Quinoa
- Soy sauce, low-sodium
- Whole-grain bread, buns, bagels, or English muffins
- Whole-grain or corn tortillas
- Whole-grain pasta

Refrigerator

- Cheese (shredded, sliced, or block), low-fat or fat-free
- Cottage cheese, low-fat or fat-free
- Eggs, whole or liquid
- Fruit, any kind
- Milk or unsweetened plant milk, low-fat or fat-free
- Salad dressing, low-fat or olive oil–based, low-sodium, if possible

- Sparkling water, sugar-free (seltzer water contains sodium, but soda water and sparkling water do not)
- Tofu
- Vegetables, any kind
- Vegetable juice, low-sodium
- Yogurt, plain unsweetened, low-fat or fat-free

Freezer

- Chicken breast, boneless, skinless
- Edamame (soybean pods), low-sodium, if possible
- Fish
- Fruit, any kind
- Shrimp
- Turkey breast, skinless
- Vegetables, any kind, plain, unseasoned and no included sauces

Herbs (dried or fresh)

- Basil
- Bay leaf
- Chives
- Cilantro or coriander
- Dill
- Italian seasoning
- Lemongrass
- Marjoram
- Mint
- Oregano
- Parsley
- Rosemary
- Sage
- Savory
- Tarragon
- Thyme

Spices

- Allspice
- Black pepper
- Cardamom
- Cayenne pepper
- Celery seed
- Chili powder
- Cinnamon
- Curry powder
- Fennel seed
- Five-spice powder
- Garlic powder (not garlic salt)
- Ginger
- Mustard seeds
- Nutmeg
- Onion powder (not onion salt)
- Paprika
- Red pepper flakes or ground chile
- Saffron
- Turmeric

Acids

- Lemon juice
- Lime juice
- Vinegar (balsamic red wine, rice, white, white wine, apple cider)

Spice Blends

Brands like Mrs. Dash have 100% salt-free spice blends for any dish. You can also make your own spice blends, such as taco seasoning, chili seasoning, Italian seasoning, and Cajun seasoning, and store them in airtight containers.

- Taco seasoning typically includes garlic powder, onion powder, chili powder, cayenne pepper or ground chile, ground cumin, dried oregano, and paprika.

- Chili seasoning usually includes primarily chili powder, with the additions of paprika, garlic powder, and onion powder.

- Italian seasoning can be purchased at the store and is usually salt-free. To make your own, combine dried basil, oregano, rosemary, parsley, and thyme.

- Cajun seasoning usually includes paprika, garlic powder, dried oregano, onion powder, black pepper, cayenne pepper, and dried thyme.

As you can see, many of these spice blends use the same herbs and spices, just in different quantities, so you can customize your blends to your taste preference.

FOODS TO TOSS, GIVE AWAY, OR LIMIT

While this is not an elimination diet, it may be easier to toss or avoid bringing certain ingredients into your kitchen to streamline your cooking process, reduce confusion, and avoid temptation. This isn't to say you can't ever enjoy these foods again—you will see occasional instances of these ingredients in the recipes to come, such as olives or turkey bacon, though they are minimal. They should only make the occasional appearance in your diet, rather than be a staple that's easily accessible in your pantry.

Pantry

- Baked goods like cakes, cookies, pastries, pie
- Boxed macaroni and cheese
- Candy
- Canned soup or chili
- Cereal bars or protein bars high in sugar
- Chips, salted

- Chocolate
- Coconut oil
- Cookies
- Creamy salad dressings and sauces
- Dry pasta and rice side dishes made with flavor packets
- Instant noodles
- Jarred olives, pickles, jalapeños
- Jarred queso
- Jarred salsa
- Jarred sauces like pasta sauce or Alfredo
- Lard
- Microwave popcorn (high in sodium and fat)

- Pudding
- Salted nuts and seeds
- Seasonings packets like taco seasoning, chili seasoning, French onion dip, ranch
- Shortening
- Snack crackers
- Soy sauce (if full sodium)
- Sugary cereals
- Toaster pastries
- Vinegar-based hot sauces (high in sodium)
- White breads, bagels, buns, English muffins

Refrigerator

- Bacon
- Beef cuts (if fatty or marbled)
- Biscuits
- Butter
- Cheese (if full-fat)
- Chicken, skin-on
- Coffee creamer
- Cookie dough
- Cream
- Cream cheese, full-fat
- Deli meat
- Dips
- Ham
- Pudding

- Sausage
- Soda (unless diet or sugar-free, which you can enjoy on a limited basis)
- Sour cream, full-fat
- Sports drinks
- Stick margarine (use of tub margarine is okay occasionally, but stick margarine should be avoided; while they look and taste similar, stick margarine is higher in trans fats)
- Turkey, skin-on
- Whole milk
- Yogurt, full-fat, sweetened

Freezer

- Cheese curds
- Chicken nuggets or tenders
- Egg rolls
- Frozen novelties
- Frozen pizza
- Ice cream
- Jalapeño poppers
- Mozzarella sticks
- Pie
- TV dinners
- Whipped cream

KITCHEN ESSENTIALS AND HELPFUL GADGETS

The recipes in this book are all simple, so you do not need any fancy or complicated equipment or gadgets. The following list includes the kitchen items that, along with your stove, oven, and microwave, will help you make a large number of the recipes in this book. I have also included items that are not necessary but will help make cooking easier for you.

- Aluminum foil
- Baking dish or casserole dish
- Baking sheet
- Blender (and/or food processor)
- Bowls, variety of sizes
- Can opener
- Cutting board
- Griddle pan or electric griddle
- Grill pan or grill (electric, charcoal, or gas)
- Knives (make sure they're sharp)
- Measuring cups and spoons (for dry and wet ingredients)
- Microwave-safe dishes
- Muffin tin, standard 12-cup
- Muffin/cupcake liners
- Parchment paper
- Pie pan
- Plastic wrap
- Saucepan with lid
- Skillet and/or sauté pan (oven-safe, if possible)
- Spatula, spoons, and ladles
- Steamer basket
- Stockpot
- Whisk
- Wooden or metal skewers
- Zip-top storage bags

Looking at the Label

The nutrition label recently got a face-lift; it looks similar to the way it did before, but the FDA has tried to make it easier to understand, while drawing extra attention to the nutrients that people look for most often, such as calories, fat, salt, and sugar.

Nutrition Facts

8 servings per container
Serving size   **1 cup (68g)**

Amount per serving
Calories   **370**

	% Daily Value*
Total Fat 5g	**7%**
Saturated Fat 1g	**3%**
Trans Fat 0g	
Cholesterol 0mg	**0%**
Sodium 150mg	**6%**
Total Carbohydrate 48g	**15%**
Dietary Fiber 5g	**14%**
Total Sugars 13g	
Includes 10g Added Sugars	**20%**
Protein 12g	
Vit. D 2mcg 10% • Calcium 210mg 20%	
Zinc 7mg 50% • Biotin 300mcg 100%	

* The % Daily Value (DV) tells you how much a nutrient in a serving of food contributes to a daily diet. 2,000 calories a day is used for general nutrition advice.

You first want to always check the **serving size**. You may think that the food you have grabbed has only 200mg of sodium, but if there are four servings per container and you eat the whole container, you have actually consumed 800mg of sodium. This same principle applies to all the numbers on the label: If you eat more than one serving, you have to multiply those numbers by the number of servings you ate.

On the DASH diet, the nutrients you want to be looking at most closely on the nutrition label are **sodium** and **fat**. A low-sodium or low-fat food will contain 5 percent or less of your daily value. A high-fat or high-sodium food will contain 20 percent or more of your daily value. On the label, fat is broken down as follows:

- **Total Fat:** This number INCLUDES the saturated and trans fats listed below it.

- **Saturated Fat:** The DASH diet promotes consuming as little saturated fat as possible.

- **Trans Fat:** The DASH diet promotes consuming as little trans fat as possible.

For example, if a product lists 10g Total Fat, 5g of which are Saturated Fat and 0g of which are Trans Fat, that means the remaining 5g are unsaturated fats (the healthy fats).

At first it may seem daunting to check the label of every food item you pick up in the store, but I promise you, it gets easier and eventually becomes second nature. You will soon know which items, brands, or labels to grab, such as "no-salt-added," and you will not have to read every label at every grocery trip.

Tips for Adjusting to a New Diet and Lifestyle

Embarking on a new diet and making major lifestyle changes is a big undertaking. You should be incredibly proud of yourself. It will take time to adjust to your new diet and active lifestyle. Along the journey, refer back to this page to give yourself a little pick-me-up, because every effort you make is progress toward helping your blood pressure. Here are my top 10 tips for success on the DASH diet.

1. **BE KIND TO YOURSELF.** First, remember that you are not your medical condition. You are not high blood pressure—you are a whole person, and just a tiny part of your life is that you have high blood pressure. You are making these dietary and lifestyle changes to treat yourself better, the way your body deserves to be treated, so do it with kindness.

2. **ACKNOWLEDGE SETBACKS.** No one is perfect. After a crazy week at work, maybe you did not cook the meals you had planned, or you ate out more times than you intended. Acknowledge that it happened, determine why it happened (to help prevent it in the future), and move forward. One "bad" meal does not mean you have to slide downhill and give up. Just focus on the next "good" meal and move forward.

3. **STICK TO THE PLAN.** The DASH diet takes all the guesswork out for you; there is no reason to reinvent the wheel. Stick to the basics provided in this book, and as you get more comfortable, you can start adding your own flair to recipes, using flavors you prefer, and customizing the diet to your unique body and needs.

4. **TRY A LITTLE BIT AT A TIME.** Implementing the entire DASH diet and lifestyle changes, like exercise, is a lot for anyone. Take it one step at a time. Try to have a week with less added salt, and then a week with less meat, and then a week with increased activity. This is a marathon, not a sprint. To make long-lasting change, you need to create new habits, which takes time, so be patient with the process.

5. **MAP OUT YOUR WEEK.** Hard work and change take planning. Sitting down once a week and writing out your schedule will allow you to slot in the meals you would like to have, which will enable you to create a detailed grocery list so you'll have all the necessary ingredients on hand.

6. **GROCERY SHOP WITH PURPOSE.** Once you have your list, stick to it. No more grabbing items that are not on the list. No last-minute chips, candy bars, and snacks. This will save you money and keep you from bringing home foods that are not on your dietary protocol.

7. **MEAL PREP (BUT NOT IN A SCARY WAY).** Meal prep has a reputation for being 20 clear containers in your fridge, each containing exact weighed portions of chicken breast, rice, and broccoli. In reality, meal prep can be as simple as making a snack to enjoy during the week or baking an extra chicken breast at dinner to shred over salad later in the week. Make use of your time and ingredients to cut down on wasted time and food waste.

8. **CHOOSE EXERCISE YOU ENJOY.** If you hate running and set out to run five days a week, I bet you probably won't do it, or at least you won't do it for the long-term. If you love coed soccer, sign up for a league and practice at the park or in your yard on non-game days. Choosing an activity you enjoy will help ensure that you stick to doing it.

9. **DON'T HESITATE TO ASK FOR HELP.** Your health care team is there to help you. Never be afraid to ask your doctor, cardiologist, or dietitian for help. There are no stupid questions, and asking your question will get you a quick, accurate answer that you can immediately apply to your life, instead of stressing, procrastinating, and feeling lost or in a rut.

10. **CREATE A SUPPORT SYSTEM FOR YOURSELF.** Having family, friends, colleagues, and even support group "strangers" on your side can be a huge help during a lifestyle change. You want people around you to encourage your progress, help keep you accountable, and make you feel good about the changes you are implementing.

DASH for the First Week

To ease you into the DASH diet, I've created an easy 7-day sample meal plan that serves one. I have utilized the weekend to prepare your snacks for the week, and have placed the quickest breakfasts and lunches during the workweek to save you time preparing in the morning. You will also have leftovers at the end of the week, which you can eat at the start of the following week to set you up for success.

I know that not everyone works a nine-to-five job, so feel free to use your days off as your prep days. This sample meal plan has a variety of flavors and ingredients, ensuring that you won't get bored during the week and giving you an opportunity to try new flavors that you may not have tried before. Embracing different flavors, herbs, and spices will make omitting salt easier.

Sample 7-Day Meal Plan

	Sunday	Monday	Tuesday	Wednesday
Breakfast	Super-Fast Breakfast Burrito (page 47)	*Leftover* Super-Fast Breakfast Burrito	Peanut Butter Banana Smoothie (page 33)	*Leftover* Super-Fast Breakfast Burrito
Lunch	Cheesy Vegetarian Rice Casserole (page 88)	*Leftover* Cheesy Vegetarian Rice Casserole	*Leftover* Lentil Soup	*Leftover* Cheesy Vegetarian Rice Casserole
Dinner	Lentil Soup (page 59)	Grilled Chicken and Vegetables in Lemon-Walnut Sauce (page 110)	*Leftover* Cheesy Vegetarian Rice Casserole	*Leftover* Grilled Chicken and Vegetables in Lemon-Walnut Sauce
Snack	Spiced Edamame (page 138) Sweet-Hot Maple Almonds (page 139) Oil and Vinegar Roasted Chickpeas (page 141)	*Leftover* Spiced Edamame	*Leftover* Sweet-Hot Maple Almonds	*Leftover* Oil and Vinegar Roasted Chickpeas

	Thursday	Friday	Saturday
Breakfast	The Green Monster (page 32)	*Leftover* Super-Fast Breakfast Burrito	Asparagus, Salmon, and Tomato Quiche (page 44)
Lunch	*Leftover* Lentil Soup	*Leftover* Grilled Chicken and Vegetables in Lemon-Walnut Sauce	*Leftover* Lentil Soup
Dinner	*Leftover* Grilled Chicken and Vegetables in Lemon-Walnut Sauce	Citrus-Kissed Flounder in Foil (page 98)	*Leftover* Citrus-Kissed Flounder in Foil
Snack	*Leftover* Spiced Edamame	*Leftover* Sweet-Hot Maple Almonds	*Leftover* Oil and Vinegar Roasted Chickpeas

About the Recipes

The recipes in this book are all balanced meals and snacks and are compliant with the blood-pressure-lowering DASH diet. They are easy, quick, and inexpensive recipes that utilize familiar, easy-to-find ingredients to make your transition into your new lifestyle as simple as possible. You will be cooking more, but these recipes will allow you to make meals all week and maintain a healthy lifestyle without spending hours in the kitchen cooking and cleaning.

The vast majority of the recipes are below 500mg of sodium per serving so you can stay within that 1,500 to 2,300mg daily range. There are a few recipes higher than 500mg per serving. These should be enjoyed occasionally and only on days that you will not exceed that upper sodium intake limit. These recipes will also have suggestions for how to lower the sodium content in the headnote or tip, if applicable.

You will also find that the recipes run the gamut from sweet to savory, tart to spicy, and everything in between, and include familiar "healthified" favorites. You will learn to prepare plant-based recipes that nourish your body and lower your blood pressure. There are plenty of fish, chicken, turkey, beef, and pork recipes as well, which exemplify heart-healthy cooking methods when following the recommended consumption of one 6-ounce serving per day.

Each recipe has labels to let you know at a glance what you can expect. These include:

ONE-POT

Create your entire dish dirtying only one pot, pan, or dish!

5 INGREDIENTS OR FEWER

Recipes that pack in big flavor with only a handful of ingredients (excluding pepper, water, and oil).

30 MINUTES OR LESS

Perfect for busy nights, or to meal prep in the morning before work.

DAIRY-FREE

These recipes do not contain dairy or dairy products.

GLUTEN-FREE

For the safety of anyone with celiac disease or a gluten sensitivity. Also, feel free to make any gluten-containing recipe gluten-free by using your favorite gluten-free bread, pasta, or flour alternative.

NUT-FREE

For the safety of anyone with a nut allergy, these recipes do not contain nuts, including tree nuts, such as coconut.

VEGETARIAN

These recipes do not contain meat or fish, but may contain dairy or eggs.

VEGAN

These recipes do not contain any animal products and are completely plant-based.

I am so excited for you to get started on the recipes in this book. I know that this book can be life-changing if you let it. You have the tools in your hands to take control of your blood pressure and own your health. You can do this. Now that you have all the technical knowledge, the whys and hows of the diet, it is time to implement change through the power of food. Bon appétit!

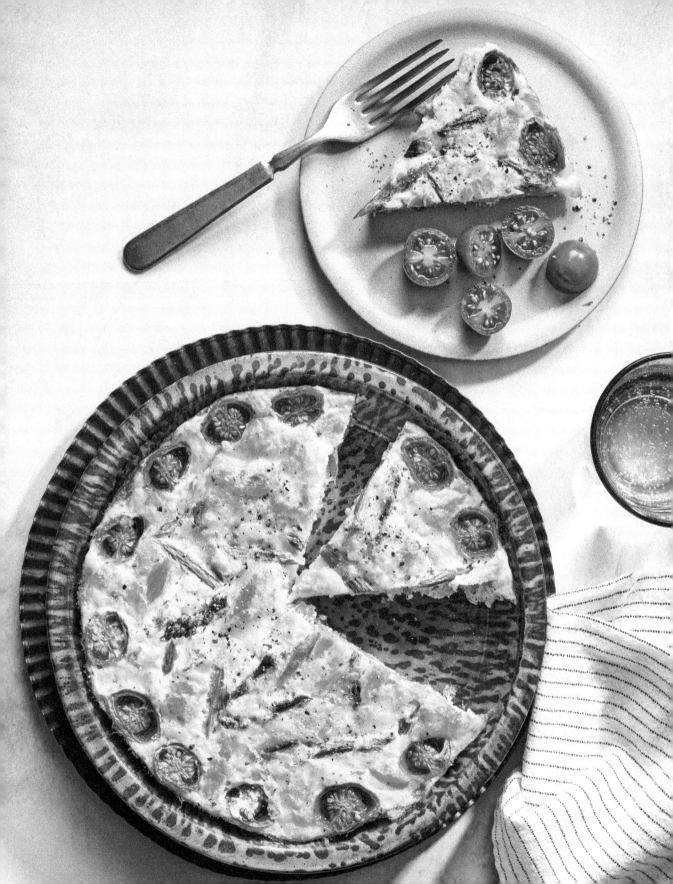

CHAPTER TWO

Breakfasts and Smoothies

ONE-POT

5 INGREDIENTS OR FEWER

30 MINUTES OR LESS

DAIRY-FREE

GLUTEN-FREE

NUT-FREE

VEGAN

The Green Monster

Serves 2 / Prep time: 15 minutes

Green smoothies are packed with nutrients as well as flavor—you won't even notice the kale hiding in this breakfast treat. The lemon and apple brighten and sweeten this smoothie, while the avocado provides important healthy fat that will keep you full all morning.

2 cups stemmed and coarsely chopped kale leaves

1 Hass avocado, pitted and chopped

1 apple, peeled, cored, and coarsely chopped

½ cup unsweetened apple juice

2 tablespoons freshly squeezed lemon juice

2 or 3 ice cubes

1. Combine the kale, avocado, and apple in a food processor or blender and process for 1 to 2 minutes, until smooth.
2. Add the apple juice, lemon juice, and ice and process again until well combined, about 1 minute more.
3. Serve immediately.

PER SERVING: Calories: 248; Total Fat: 15g; Saturated Fat: 2g; Cholesterol: 0mg; Sodium: 17mg; Potassium: 742mg; Carbohydrates: 31g; Fiber: 10g; Sugars: 17g; Protein: 3g

Peanut Butter Banana Smoothie

Serves 1 / Prep time: 10 minutes

This smoothie provides an excellent balance of nutrients to start your day off right. Protein and healthy fat from the peanut butter will keep you full and energized, while the banana provides just enough sweetness to satisfy that morning sweet tooth. You can use a plant-based milk in place of the skim milk and achieve the same creamy results.

1 cup skim milk
½ cup sliced banana
4 ice cubes
1 tablespoon unsalted natural
   peanut butter

1 teaspoon unsweetened cacao powder
   (optional)
½ teaspoon vanilla extract

1. Combine the milk, banana, ice, peanut butter, cacao powder (if using), and vanilla in a blender and blend for about 1 minute, until smooth.
2. Pour into a glass and enjoy immediately.

SUBSTITUTION TIP: You can use any unsalted nut or seed butter you prefer in this recipe.

PER SERVING: Calories: 271; Total Fat: 11g; Saturated Fat: 3g; Cholesterol: 12mg; Sodium: 111mg; Potassium: 727mg; Carbohydrates: 33g; Fiber: 3g; Sugars: 24g; Protein: 13g

Peach and Walnut Breakfast Salad

Serves 1 / Prep time: 10 minutes

Cottage cheese is a protein powerhouse that is delicious in sweet or savory recipes. This breakfast salad is sure to become a household favorite with its brightness from the peaches, lemon, and mint, crunch from the walnuts, and sweetness from the honey. Satisfaction guaranteed!

½ cup low-fat or fat-free cottage cheese
1 ripe peach, pitted and sliced
¼ cup chopped raw unsalted walnuts, toasted

1 teaspoon honey
1 tablespoon chopped fresh mint
Pinch of grated lemon zest

1. Spoon the cottage cheese into a small bowl and top with the peach slices and walnuts.
2. Drizzle with the honey, then top with the mint and lemon zest. Serve.

PREP TIP: To toast the walnuts, place them on a rimmed baking sheet in a single layer. Bake at 350°F for 7 to 10 minutes, stirring or shaking the pan frequently to brown the nuts evenly. Be sure to watch the walnuts the entire time to prevent burning.

PER SERVING: Calories: 356; Total Fat: 21g; Saturated Fat: 3g; Cholesterol: 5mg; Sodium: 321mg; Potassium: 541mg; Carbohydrates: 28g; Fiber: 5g; Sugars: 22g; Protein: 20g

Coconut Rice Pudding

Serves 4 / Prep time: 5 minutes / Cook time: 25 minutes, plus 10 minutes to rest

Rice pudding is a dish that is found in countless cultures worldwide. Most rice puddings share the hallmarks of rice, milk, spices, and sweetener. It is most commonly eaten as breakfast or dessert. This breakfast variation is loaded with antioxidant-rich dried cherries and healthy fat and protein from the nuts.

1 tablespoon orange-infused olive oil or plain olive oil
1 cup cooked long-grain rice
1 cup canned lite coconut milk
1 cinnamon stick
1 teaspoon vanilla extract

½ cup skim milk
½ cup unsweetened dried cherries
½ cup raw unsalted pecans or almonds, toasted
Pinch ground nutmeg

1. In a medium sauté pan, heat the oil over medium heat until warmed. Add the cooked rice, coconut milk, cinnamon stick, and vanilla and stir to combine.
2. Bring to a simmer, then reduce the heat to low and cook, partially covered, until the coconut milk is absorbed, about 20 minutes. Remove from the heat.
3. Add the skim milk, cherries, pecans, and nutmeg. Cover and let rest for 10 minutes before serving. Add more milk if needed to achieve the desired consistency. Store leftovers in an airtight container in the refrigerator for 3 to 4 days.

PREP TIP: Rice keeps well in the refrigerator, so any time you have leftover rice, simply store it in an airtight container or bag in the fridge so you can make this recipe in a fraction of the time. You can also use ground cinnamon, if you do not have a cinnamon stick on hand.

PER SERVING: Calories: 261; Total Fat: 17g; Saturated Fat: 8g; Cholesterol: 2mg; Sodium: 20mg; Potassium: 239mg; Carbohydrates: 24g; Fiber: 2g; Sugars: 9g; Protein: 4g

Savory Oat Bowl

Serves 2 / Prep time: 10 minutes / Cook time: 20 minutes

Eating oatmeal in a savory capacity may sound new and strange, but trust me, it is delightful. Think about oats as a neutral flavor base similar to rice or flour. You will love the chew of the steel-cut oats combined with the crunchy fresh veggies and herbs. This recipe is a nice intro to savory oatmeal, so feel free to get creative and jazz yours up with leftover vegetables, spices, and even beans!

1 cup water
½ cup steel-cut oats
1 large tomato, chopped
1 medium cucumber, peeled, seeded, and chopped

1 tablespoon olive oil
Chopped fresh flat-leaf parsley or mint, for garnish
Freshly ground black pepper

1. In a medium saucepan, combine the water and oats and bring to a boil over high heat.
2. Cook, stirring continuously, until the water is absorbed, about 15 minutes.
3. To serve, divide the oatmeal between two bowls and top with the tomatoes and cucumber. Drizzle with the oil, then top with the parsley. Season with pepper and serve.

PREP TIP: To make overnight oats for a fast grab-and-go breakfast option, combine old-fashioned oats and water in a lidded container, mix well, seal, and refrigerate overnight. The next morning, heat before adding the toppings, or enjoy chilled.

PER SERVING: Calories: 269; Total Fat: 10g; Saturated Fat: 2g; Cholesterol: 0mg; Sodium: 9mg; Potassium: 447mg; Carbohydrates: 38g; Fiber: 7g; Sugars: 5g; Protein: 9g

Date-Sweetened Chocolate Oatmeal

Serves 2 / Prep time: 5 minutes / Cook time: 10 minutes

Dates are a wonderful natural sweetener. They contain the sweetness you crave along with the added nutritional benefits of essential vitamins and minerals, antioxidants, and fiber. Adding a couple of chopped dates to your oatmeal is a great alternative to brown sugar or honey.

1 cup skim milk

1 cup water

1 cup old-fashioned oats

¼ cup pitted dates (2 to 3 dates), chopped

2 tablespoons unsweetened cacao powder

1. In a medium saucepan, combine the milk, water, oats, dates, and cacao powder and heat over medium heat until almost boiling.
2. Cook, stirring constantly, for about 2 minutes, until the mixture is creamy. Serve hot.

SUBSTITUTION TIP: Make this recipe vegan by using a plant-based milk. Alternatively, add your favorite unsweetened protein powder for added protein, if desired.

PER SERVING: Calories: 269; Total Fat: 5g; Saturated Fat: 2g; Cholesterol: 6mg; Sodium: 58mg; Potassium: 586mg; Carbohydrates: 50g; Fiber: 7g; Sugars: 19g; Protein: 11g

Blueberry and Quinoa Cereal

Serves 2 / Prep time: 5 minutes / Cook time: 20 minutes

Similar to oatmeal, quinoa is another food that can be the star of both sweet and savory dishes. Classified as a whole grain, quinoa is loaded with plant-based protein as well as fiber, essential for heart health and healthy digestion. This quinoa cereal is hearty, warming, and filling, just what you need to start your day off right.

1 teaspoon canola oil
¾ cup quinoa, rinsed and drained
½ teaspoon ground nutmeg
1 cup water

2 cups fresh blueberries
½ cup unsweetened vanilla almond milk
1 teaspoon vanilla extract

1. In a heavy medium sauté pan or skillet, heat the oil over medium-high heat. Add the quinoa and nutmeg and cook, stirring frequently, for 2 minutes.
2. Add the water and simmer, uncovered, for 10 minutes, or until the quinoa is still slightly crunchy.
3. Add the blueberries, almond milk, and vanilla and stir well. Simmer for 4 minutes, ladle into bowls, and serve warm.

INGREDIENT TIP: You can use thawed frozen blueberries in place of fresh.

PER SERVING: Calories: 368; Total Fat: 8g; Saturated Fat: 1g; Cholesterol: 0mg; Sodium: 26mg; Potassium: 553mg; Carbohydrates: 64g; Fiber: 8g; Sugars: 15g; Protein: 12g

Blueberry Oat Pancakes

Serves 4 / Prep time: 5 minutes / Cook time: 25 minutes

Just because you're eating a low-sodium, heart-healthy diet doesn't mean you have to forgo your morning pancakes. High in fiber and big on protein, these pancakes are perfect breakfast fuel that will get you to lunch before you know it. If you want to knock down the sodium content further, substitute applesauce for the yogurt.

1½ cups water
½ cup steel-cut oats
1 cup whole-wheat flour
1 cup low-fat milk
½ cup plain low-fat Greek yogurt
1 large egg

1 teaspoon vanilla extract
½ teaspoon baking powder
½ teaspoon baking soda
1 cup blueberries, fresh or thawed frozen
2 teaspoons canola oil, divided
½ cup pure maple syrup (optional)

1. In a medium saucepan, combine the water and oats. Bring the mixture to a boil over medium heat, then reduce the heat to low. Simmer, stirring often, for 15 minutes. Remove the pot from the heat and set aside.
2. Meanwhile, in a medium bowl, combine the flour, milk, yogurt, egg, vanilla, baking powder, and baking soda. Mix until just smooth. Stir the oatmeal to loosen it up, then mix it into the batter along with the blueberries.
3. On a griddle or in a skillet, heat ½ teaspoon of the oil over medium heat. Working in batches, use a measuring cup to pour about ¼ cup of batter per pancake onto the griddle. Cook until the batter bubbles on top and the pancakes are golden on the bottom, 2 to 3 minutes. Flip the pancakes and cook for another 2 minutes. Transfer the pancakes to a warm plate and cover with foil or a clean kitchen towel to keep warm.
4. Repeat until all the batter is used up, adding more oil to the pan as needed. Divide the batch of pancakes into four equal portions and serve with the maple syrup on the side, if desired.

PER SERVING: Calories: 256; Total Fat: 7g; Saturated Fat: 2g; Cholesterol: 53mg; Sodium: 227mg; Potassium: 376mg; Carbohydrates: 40g; Fiber: 5g; Sugars: 9g; Protein: 11g

Spring Vegetable Frittata

Serves 2 / Prep time: 5 minutes / Cook time: 15 minutes

This egg white frittata starts your day with lean protein, healthy fat, and a hearty serving of vegetables. I love moving vegetables from the dinner plate to the breakfast plate because they are nutritious and filling—a perfect way to head into the day, ready to tackle anything. Feel free to substitute any vegetables you like (including leftover vegetables) in this recipe.

4 large egg whites, or ½ cup liquid egg whites

1 teaspoon skim milk

1 tablespoon olive oil

1 cup chopped spinach

4 asparagus spears, cooked and chopped

¼ red bell pepper, chopped

Freshly ground black pepper

¼ cup crumbled goat cheese

1. Preheat the broiler with a rack in the middle position. In a small bowl, beat the egg whites with the skim milk until just combined.
2. In a small oven-safe sauté pan or skillet, heat the oil over medium-high heat, then add the egg whites.
3. Spread the spinach on top of the egg whites in an even layer, then top with the asparagus and bell pepper. Season with black pepper to taste. Reduce the heat to medium and cook for 3 minutes, or until the bottom of the egg whites is firm and the vegetables are tender.
4. Top with the goat cheese and transfer the skillet to the middle rack under the broiler. Broil for 3 minutes, or until the egg whites are firm in the middle and the cheese has melted.
5. Slice into wedges and serve immediately.

INGREDIENT TIP: Although asparagus is available all year, it is most nutritious in the early spring when it is in season. In the fall, substitute cubed cooked butternut squash or cooked Brussels sprouts. Jarred or thawed frozen vegetables work equally well in this recipe; just make sure they don't have added salt.

PER SERVING: Calories: 146; Total Fat: 10g; Saturated Fat: 3g; Cholesterol: 7mg; Sodium: 192mg; Potassium: 294mg; Carbohydrates: 3g; Fiber: 1g; Sugars: 2g; Protein: 11g

Mediterranean Spinach Omelet

Serves 1 / Prep time: 5 minutes / Cook time: 15 minutes

Mediterranean dishes are wonderfully heart healthy, utilizing olive oil, tons of vegetables, and lean dairy. The flavors in this omelet are sure to excite your senses, invoking your savory palate to fill you up for a busy day. Bulk up this omelet by adding any veggies you prefer.

1 teaspoon olive oil
½ cup sliced button or cremini
  mushrooms
1 cup chopped spinach
1 large egg

2 large egg whites, or ¼ cup liquid egg
  whites
2 tablespoons crumbled feta cheese
1 teaspoon chopped fresh oregano
Freshly ground black pepper

1. In a medium sauté pan or skillet, heat the oil over medium heat. Add the mushrooms and sauté until they release their liquid, about 4 minutes.
2. Add the spinach and cook until it wilts, 2 to 3 minutes. Transfer the mixture to a small bowl, cover to keep it warm, and set aside.
3. Pour the egg and egg whites into the same skillet, mix well, and cook over medium heat until the outer edges set. Use a spatula to loosen the edges from the pan. Lift the edges at several points around the pan and tilt the pan so the uncooked egg runs under the cooked egg.
4. When the eggs are mostly set, 2 to 3 minutes, scatter the feta and sautéed spinach and mushrooms over the top. Sprinkle on the oregano and season with pepper. Fold the omelet in half and cook for 1 minute.
5. Serve immediately.

PER SERVING: Calories: 194; Total Fat: 14g; Saturated Fat: 5g; Cholesterol: 203mg; Sodium: 320mg; Potassium: 422mg; Carbohydrates: 4g; Fiber: 1g; Sugars: 2g; Protein: 14g

ONE-POT

30 MINUTES OR LESS

GLUTEN-FREE

NUT-FREE

VEGETARIAN

Sweet Potato and Brussels Sprout Hash with Soft-Boiled Eggs

Serves 4 / Prep time: 5 minutes / Cook time: 20 minutes

Orange-fleshed sweet potatoes, which are full of beta-carotene and fiber, are much more nutritious than their white-potato counterparts. This breakfast is full of healthy fat and protein from the eggs, complex carbohydrates from the potatoes, and fiber from the vegetables to keep you full and satiated all morning long. If you don't like a runny yolk, cook the eggs any way you prefer.

2 tablespoons olive oil
2 garlic cloves, minced
½ red onion, diced
2 sweet potatoes, peeled and diced
8 ounces Brussels sprouts, trimmed and sliced crosswise

1 teaspoon minced fresh thyme or dried
½ teaspoon freshly ground black pepper
4 large eggs

1. Fill a medium saucepan with about 4 inches of water and bring to a boil over high heat.
2. Meanwhile, in a large sauté pan or skillet, heat the oil over medium heat. Add the garlic and cook, stirring, for 1 minute. Add the onion and cook, stirring occasionally, until it begins to soften, 2 to 3 minutes.
3. Increase the heat to medium-high and add the sweet potatoes. Cook, stirring occasionally, until the sweet potatoes begin to brown, about 8 minutes.
4. Add the Brussels sprouts and cook for 4 to 5 minutes, until they begin to brown. Season with the thyme and pepper.
5. When the water in the saucepan is boiling, carefully add the eggs. Reduce the heat to low and simmer for 6 minutes. Drain the eggs and rinse under cold water.
6. Divide the hash evenly among four serving plates. Carefully peel the eggs and place one on top of each serving of hash. Serve immediately. Store leftover hash and eggs (in their shells) in an airtight container in the refrigerator for up to 3 days.

PER SERVING: Calories: 219; Total Fat: 12g; Saturated Fat: 3g; Cholesterol: 136mg; Sodium: 122mg; Potassium: 536mg; Carbohydrates: 20g; Fiber: 4g; Sugars: 5g; Protein: 9g

Egg Sausage Sandwich

Serves 4 / Prep time: 10 minutes / Cook time: 20 minutes

Making your own sausage is simple and allows you to eliminate most of the sodium. Pork is often associated with being high in fat and salt, but lean ground pork and lean pork chops are excellent protein choices on the DASH diet. The herbs and spices give it plenty of flavor without added salt. Enjoy this breakfast sandwich "open-faced" to lower the sodium per serving, if desired.

1 pound lean ground pork
1 teaspoon dried sage
½ teaspoon ground white pepper
½ teaspoon dried marjoram
½ teaspoon ground ginger
⅛ teaspoon ground nutmeg
Nonstick cooking spray

4 large egg whites, or ½ cup liquid egg whites
4 whole-grain English muffins, split
4 low-fat Cheddar cheese slices
4 tomato slices
4 avocado slices

1. In a large bowl, combine the pork, sage, white pepper, marjoram, ginger, and nutmeg and mix well. Form into four patties.
2. Heat a nonstick griddle over medium heat. Spray the griddle with cooking spray. Add the patties to pan, and cook until well browned and cooked through, about 8 minutes per side.
3. Meanwhile, spray a small microwave-safe bowl with cooking spray. Add the egg whites and microwave on high until cooked through, about 2 minutes. Cook for an additional 30 seconds, if needed.
4. While the eggs cook, toast the English muffins. Cut the cooked eggs into four pieces and remove from the bowl.
5. Place the English muffins on a plate and layer the cheese, tomato, avocado, sausage patties, and egg onto the muffins. Serve. To store leftover sandwiches, omit the tomato and avocado, wrap individually in foil, and store in an airtight zip-top bag in the refrigerator for up to 3 days or in the freezer for up to 1 month.

PER SERVING: Calories: 382; Total Fat: 12g; Saturated Fat: 4g; Cholesterol: 73mg; Sodium: 618mg; Potassium: 726mg; Carbohydrates: 31g; Fiber: 6g; Sugars: 6g; Protein: 41g

Asparagus, Salmon, and Tomato Quiche

Serves 8 / Prep time: 10 minutes / Cook time: 30 minutes

You may be asking, "Fish for breakfast?" YES, absolutely! Fish (like salmon) is one of the smartest protein choices you can make due to its high levels of omega-3 fatty acids, literally fueling your day with brain food. And as a bonus, because salmon is delicious any time of day, this recipe would be perfect not only for breakfast but also for brunch, lunch, or dinner.

Nonstick cooking spray
1 tablespoon canola oil
1 cup chopped onion
6 asparagus spears, chopped into ½-inch
  pieces
8 large egg whites, or 1 cup liquid egg
  whites

½ cup shredded low-fat mozzarella
  cheese
¼ teaspoon freshly ground black or white
  pepper
4 ounces smoked salmon, chopped
½ cup halved cherry tomatoes

1. Preheat the oven to 350°F. Coat a pie pan with cooking spray.
2. In a medium sauté pan, heat the oil over medium-high heat. Add the onion and asparagus and sauté until the onion begins to caramelize, about 8 minutes.
3. In a large bowl, mix the egg whites, cheese, and pepper. Gently mix in the asparagus and onion mixture as well as the salmon.
4. Pour the egg mixture into the pie pan. Place the tomatoes in a circle around the outer edge of the egg mixture.
5. Bake for 30 minutes, or until the eggs are set at the center. Let rest for 5 minutes before serving. Store leftovers in an airtight container in the refrigerator for up to 3 days.

SERVING TIP: This quiche is delicious leftover and is tasty cold or at room temperature.

PER SERVING: Calories: 83; Total Fat: 4g; Saturated Fat: 1g; Cholesterol: 8mg; Sodium: 388mg; Potassium: 163mg; Carbohydrates: 3g; Fiber: 1g; Sugars: 2g; Protein: 8g

Open-Faced Turkey Bacon and Tomato Sandwiches

Serves 2 / Prep time: 10 minutes / Cook time: 10 minutes

Though you shouldn't eat it every morning, low-sodium turkey bacon can be enjoyed in moderation. This sandwich will satisfy any occasional bacon-and-egg cravings beautifully without compromising your diet or your health. Add butter lettuce, romaine lettuce, or spinach for a breakfast BLT.

4 low-sodium turkey bacon slices
2 slices whole-grain bread
½ teaspoon canola oil

4 large eggs
4 thin slices tomato
2 thin slices reduced-fat Swiss cheese

1. Cook the bacon in the microwave according to the package instructions and set aside. Meanwhile, toast the bread in a toaster until lightly golden. Set aside.
2. In a medium sauté pan or skillet, heat the oil over medium heat. Add the eggs and cook for 1 minute to allow whites to begin setting, then pierce the yolks several times. Cook for about 5 minutes more, until the yolks are cooked through. Transfer the eggs to a plate or cutting board, add the tomato slices to the hot pan, and turn off the heat to warm through.
3. Preheat the broiler. Line a small baking sheet with foil.
4. Place the toast on the baking sheet and add two tomato slices to each piece of toast. Top each piece of toast with two eggs and one slice of cheese. Broil for 1 to 2 minutes, until the cheese is bubbling. Serve hot.

PER SERVING: Calories: 333; Total Fat: 16g; Saturated Fat: 5g; Cholesterol: 399mg; Sodium: 489mg; Potassium: 390mg; Carbohydrates: 17g; Fiber: 2g; Sugars: 3g; Protein: 28g

Ranchero Tortilla Cups

Serves 6 / Prep time: 10 minutes / Cook time: 17 minutes

If you have a taste for a south-of-the-border breakfast, this recipe will fit the bill. It looks like something you took a lot of care to prepare, but it actually takes just minutes. This recipe serves six, so it's a good one for weekend guests or to meal prep for a week of grab-and-go breakfasts. Use corn tortillas instead of flour tortillas to make these gluten-free.

1 tablespoon olive oil, divided
6 (6-inch) flour tortillas
1 (15-ounce) can no-salt-added black beans, drained and rinsed
¾ cup salsa
6 large eggs

½ cup shredded reduced-fat Mexican-style cheese blend
¼ cup low-fat or nonfat sour cream
Fresh flat-leaf parsley, chopped, for garnish

1. Preheat the oven to 375°F. Lightly grease six cups of a muffin tin with oil.
2. Use the remaining oil to lightly coat one side of each tortilla. Press each tortilla, oil-side down, into a prepared muffin cup.
3. Layer the black beans in each tortilla cup, followed by the salsa. Crack 1 egg into each, then top with the shredded cheese.
4. Bake for 15 to 17 minutes, until eggs are cooked through and set.
5. Transfer each cup to a plate and top with a small dollop of the sour cream. Garnish with parsley and serve. Store leftovers in an airtight container in the refrigerator for 3 to 4 days.

SUBSTITUTION TIP: To lower the sodium content of this recipe, make your own salsa (see page 76) instead of using store-bought salsa or substitute the salsa with ¾ cup of diced tomatoes.

PER SERVING: Calories: 305; Total Fat: 13g; Saturated Fat: 4g; Cholesterol: 195mg; Sodium: 533mg; Potassium: 385mg; Carbohydrates: 32g; Fiber: 5g; Sugars: 2g; Protein: 16g

Super-Fast Breakfast Burrito

Serves 4 / Prep time: 5 minutes / Cook time: 5 minutes

Making eggs in the microwave is a quick, mess-free way to get a healthy breakfast on the table in just minutes. Black beans add extra fiber and protein to this flavorful breakfast wrap. Use any type of onion you prefer or have on hand instead of the scallions here, and make your own salsa (see page 76) instead of using diced tomatoes.

4 large egg whites, or ½ cup liquid
   egg whites
2 large eggs
¼ cup low-fat milk
⅛ teaspoon freshly ground black pepper
4 whole-wheat tortillas
½ cup shredded reduced-fat sharp
   Cheddar cheese

1 cup no-salt-added canned black beans,
   drained and rinsed
¼ cup chopped scallions (white and
   green parts)
½ cup diced tomatoes or homemade
   salsa (page 76)
¼ cup nonfat sour cream

1. In a microwave-safe dish, whisk together the egg whites, eggs, milk, and pepper. Cook in the microwave on high for 3 minutes. Remove the dish from the microwave and stir. Microwave for 1 additional minute, or until the eggs are set.
2. Place 1 tortilla on each of four microwave-safe plates. Divide the egg mixture evenly among the tortillas. Top each with one-quarter of the cheese, beans, and scallions.
3. Wrap the burritos up and microwave for 30 seconds. Serve immediately, topped with tomatoes and sour cream. Wrap leftover burritos in plastic wrap and store in the refrigerator for up to 3 days.

PER SERVING: Calories: 281; Total Fat: 10g; Saturated Fat: 5g; Cholesterol: 102mg; Sodium: 673mg; Potassium: 519mg; Carbohydrates: 32g; Fiber: 8g; Sugars: 3g; Protein: 20g

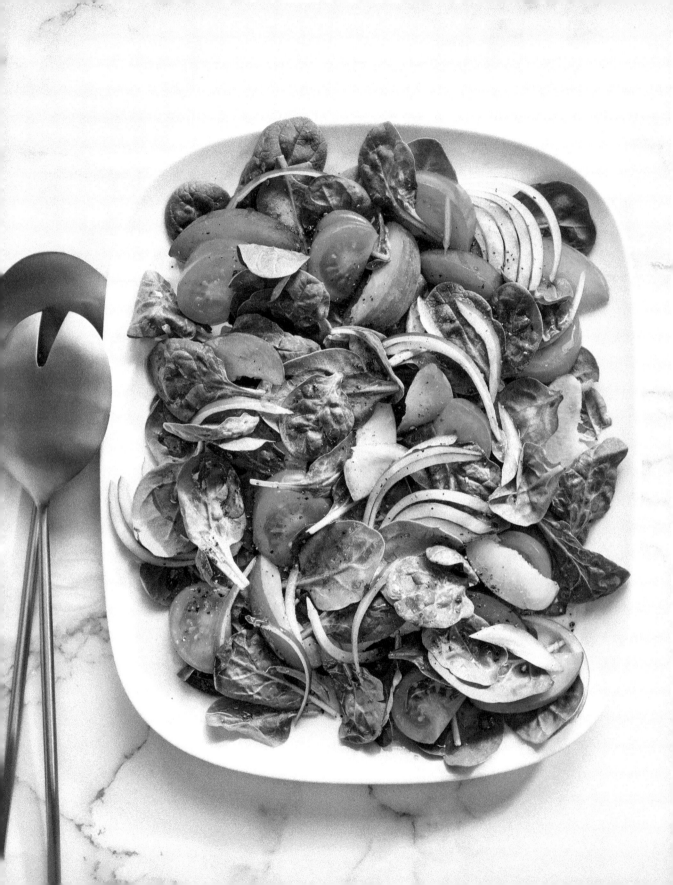

CHAPTER THREE

Salads, Soups, and Sides

ONE-POT

5 INGREDIENTS OR FEWER

30 MINUTES OR LESS

DAIRY-FREE

GLUTEN-FREE

NUT-FREE

VEGAN

Peachy Tomato Salad

Serves 2 / Prep time: 10 minutes

This salad brings me straight to summertime. I close my eyes and I can feel the sun on my face at a backyard cookout. The crisp, sweet, and bright flavors of this salad make it the perfect appetizer or side dish to a lean-protein main dish. Add low-fat mozzarella balls for more protein and flavor.

4 cups baby spinach
2 ripe peaches, pitted and sliced
   into wedges
2 ripe tomatoes, cut into wedges
½ red onion, thinly sliced

Freshly ground black pepper
3 tablespoons olive oil
1 tablespoon freshly squeezed
   lemon juice

1. In a large bowl, toss the spinach, peaches, tomatoes, and onion.
2. Season with pepper to taste. Add the oil and lemon juice and gently toss.
3. Serve at room temperature.

PER SERVING: Calories: 286; Total Fat: 21g; Saturated Fat: 3g; Cholesterol: 0mg; Sodium: 55mg; Potassium: 960mg; Carbohydrates: 24g; Fiber: 6g; Sugars: 17g; Protein: 4g

Herbed Potato Salad with Green Goddess Dressing

Serves 4 / Prep time: 25 minutes / Cook time: 5 minutes

This salad plays up the fresh flavors of herbs. Adjust the seasonings to your taste or substitute any other soft herbs. If avocados are out of season, vacuum-packed avocado or guacamole will do. If the yogurt you have isn't tangy enough for your taste, add up to a tablespoon of white vinegar to it.

2 pounds waxy potatoes, cut into 1-inch pieces
½ cup low-fat plain yogurt
1 avocado, pitted and peeled
¼ cup coarsely chopped fresh basil
½ cucumber, peeled, seeded, and chopped

¼ cup minced fresh dill
¼ cup minced fresh flat-leaf parsley
¼ cup minced fresh mint
2 scallions (white and green parts), minced
¼ teaspoon freshly ground black or white pepper

1. Put the potatoes in a large saucepan or Dutch oven and cover with water by 1 inch. Bring to a boil over high heat, then turn off the heat. Let the potatoes stand for 5 minutes, then drain and allow to cool.
2. Meanwhile, in a food processor, combine the yogurt, avocado, and basil. Process for 2 minutes, or until smooth. Pour the dressing into a large salad bowl.
3. Add the potatoes, cucumber, dill, parsley, mint, scallions, and pepper. Toss to combine and serve. Store leftovers in an airtight container in the refrigerator for up to 3 days.

PER SERVING: Calories: 287; Total Fat: 8g; Saturated Fat: 1g; Cholesterol: 0mg; Sodium: 45mg; Potassium: 1402mg; Carbohydrates: 49g; Fiber: 9g; Sugars: 5g; Protein: 8g

Arugula Artichoke Salad

Serves 6 / Prep time: 15 minutes

Arugula, also known as rocket, is a dark leafy green that has a peppery bite. It's very flavorful and has plenty of vitamins A, C, and K, as well as vital phytonutrients. Make this salad with the sweetest cherry tomatoes you can find.

¼ cup olive oil
2 tablespoons balsamic vinegar
1 teaspoon Dijon mustard
1 garlic clove, minced
6 cups arugula

1 cup cherry tomatoes, halved
6 oil-packed artichoke hearts, sliced
6 olives, pitted and chopped
4 fresh basil leaves, thinly sliced

1. In a small bowl, whisk together the oil, vinegar, Dijon, and garlic until smooth and emulsified. Set aside.
2. In a large bowl, toss the arugula, tomatoes, artichokes, and olives together.
3. Drizzle the salad with the dressing, garnish with the basil, and serve. Store leftovers in an airtight container in the refrigerator for 1 to 2 days.

SERVING TIP: Top this salad with roasted chicken, grilled shrimp, or another protein, if desired.

PER SERVING: Calories: 133; Total Fat: 12g; Saturated Fat: 2g; Cholesterol: 0mg; Sodium: 75mg; Potassium: 217mg; Carbohydrates: 6g; Fiber: 3g; Sugars: 2g; Protein: 2g

Asparagus and Edamame Salad

Serves 4 / Prep time: 10 minutes

Asparagus is a great source of fiber, antioxidants, vitamins, and minerals. And edamame is loaded with fiber, vitamins, and minerals, as well as protein.

FOR THE DRESSING

Grated zest and juice of 1 lemon

1 tablespoon white wine vinegar

1 teaspoon Dijon mustard

1 teaspoon honey

¼ teaspoon freshly ground black pepper

3 tablespoons olive oil

FOR THE SALAD

1 pound asparagus, trimmed and very thinly sliced on the diagonal

2 cups frozen shelled edamame, thawed

½ bunch radishes, thinly sliced

6 handfuls arugula

¼ cup grated reduced-fat Parmesan cheese, for garnish

TO MAKE THE DRESSING

1. In a small bowl, whisk together the lemon zest and juice, vinegar, mustard, honey, and pepper.
2. Whisk in the oil until the dressing is well combined and emulsified. Set aside.

TO MAKE THE SALAD

3. In a medium bowl, combine the asparagus, edamame, and radishes. Drizzle about three-quarters of the dressing over and toss well to coat.
4. In a medium bowl, combine the arugula with the remaining dressing and toss to coat.
5. Arrange the arugula on four salad plates, top with the asparagus mixture, and serve immediately, garnished with the Parmesan. Store leftovers in an airtight container in the refrigerator for 1 to 2 days.

PER SERVING: Calories: 239; Total Fat: 16g; Saturated Fat: 3g; Cholesterol: 6mg; Sodium: 125mg; Potassium: 681mg; Carbohydrates: 16g; Fiber: 7g; Sugars: 6g; Protein: 13g

Tuscan Kale Salad Massaged with Roasted Garlic

Serves 4 / Prep time: 10 minutes / Cook time: 45 minutes

Even though kale is extremely good for you—it's absolutely packed with the antioxidant vitamins A, C, and K—this leafy green can be tough. However, it is delicious when prepared properly. This salad uses Tuscan kale (also known as lacinato or dinosaur kale) rather than the more familiar curly variety because Tuscan kale is more tender, especially when raw.

FOR THE DRESSING

1 whole garlic head, unpeeled but with loose, papery skin removed

1 tablespoon plus 2½ teaspoons olive oil, divided

2 tablespoons freshly squeezed lemon juice

1 tablespoon low-sodium soy sauce

½ teaspoon freshly ground black pepper

FOR THE SALAD

1 red onion, thinly sliced into rings, rings separated

1 tablespoon olive oil

4 bunches Tuscan kale (about 1½ pounds)

½ cup unsweetened dried cranberries

¼ cup chopped raw unsalted hazelnuts

TO MAKE THE DRESSING

1. Preheat the oven to 500°F.
2. Cut off the pointy end of the garlic head so the tips of the cloves are sliced open.
3. Coat the outside of the head with ½ teaspoon of the oil. Put the head on a piece of foil, gather the edges of the foil together, and pinch to create a tight packet.
4. Roast the garlic until it is very soft, about 45 minutes. Remove it from the oven and set aside to cool.
5. When the garlic is cool enough to handle, hold the head over a medium bowl and use your hands to squeeze the head and push the garlic flesh out of the skins. Break the head apart and squeeze any cloves that still contain flesh.
6. Mash the flesh with the back of a spoon, then add the lemon juice, soy sauce, pepper, and remaining 1 tablespoon plus 2 teaspoons oil. Whisk the dressing until thoroughly combined.

TO MAKE THE SALAD

7. Meanwhile, in a medium bowl, toss the onion rings with the oil and spread on a baking sheet.

8. When the garlic has roasted for 30 minutes, place the onions in the oven and roast, stirring once or twice, until the onions are soft and golden brown, about 15 minutes. Remove the onions from the oven and set aside to cool.

9. While the onions and garlic cook, cut the tough stem out of each kale leaf, about two-thirds of the way up the leaf.

10. Working in batches, roll together several leaves at a time like a cigar and cut crosswise to make ½-inch-wide strips. You should have about 6 cups of kale strips.

11. In a large bowl, toss the kale with the dressing. Use your hands to rub the dressing into the kale; it will soften, shrink slightly, and turn a brighter green.

12. Add the cranberries, hazelnuts, and cooled onion and toss to coat. Store leftovers in an airtight container in the refrigerator for 2 to 3 days.

PER SERVING: Calories: 253; Total Fat: 15g; Saturated Fat: 2g; Cholesterol: 0mg; Sodium: 195mg; Potassium: 966mg; Carbohydrates: 27g; Fiber: 8g; Sugars: 11g; Protein: 9g

Spinach Waldorf Salad

Serves 2 / Prep time: 15 minutes

This crisp, refreshing salad is a crunchy, decadent dish that will make you rethink salads. The fat content may seem high, but most of the fat in this salad comes from heart-healthy walnuts, avocado, and olive oil.

FOR THE SALAD

2 low-sodium turkey bacon slices

4 cups spinach

1 cup chopped apples

¼ cup raw unsalted walnuts, chopped

1 tablespoon chopped scallion (white and green parts)

1 tablespoon unsweetened dried cranberries

FOR THE DRESSING

¼ cup low-fat plain Greek yogurt

1 tablespoon smashed avocado

1 tablespoon olive oil

1 teaspoon freshly squeezed lemon juice

1 teaspoon minced fresh basil

1 teaspoon minced fresh flat-leaf parsley

½ teaspoon chopped scallion (green part only)

½ teaspoon minced garlic

TO MAKE THE SALAD

1. Cook the bacon in the microwave according to the package instructions. Allow to cool, then chop.
2. In a large bowl, toss the spinach, bacon, apples, walnuts, scallion, and cranberries together and divide into 2-cup portions.

TO MAKE THE DRESSING

3. In a small bowl, combine the yogurt, avocado, oil, and lemon juice. Mix well.
4. Add the basil, parsley, scallion, and garlic. Drizzle 1 tablespoon of the dressing over each salad and serve.

PER SERVING: Calories: 254; Total Fat: 20g; Saturated Fat: 3g; Cholesterol: 10mg; Sodium: 176mg; Potassium: 620mg; Carbohydrates: 15g; Fiber: 4g; Sugars: 9g; Protein: 8g

Cold Cucumber Soup

Serves 4 / Prep time: 15 minutes, plus 2 hours to chill

Cucumber soup is a Polish staple, featuring tart flavors and a creamy consistency that is delightful on a warm day. This soup pairs perfectly with a lean protein main dish, a salad, and especially a hearty sandwich, or can be enjoyed alone as a refreshing chilled soup.

2 seedless cucumbers, peeled and cut into chunks
2 cups low-fat plain Greek yogurt
½ cup finely chopped fresh mint
2 garlic cloves, peeled

2 cups low-sodium vegetable broth
1 tablespoon chopped fresh dill
1 tablespoon low-sodium tomato paste
Freshly ground black pepper

1. In a food processor or blender, combine the cucumber, yogurt, mint, and garlic and puree.
2. Add the broth, dill, tomato paste, and pepper and process to incorporate.
3. Refrigerate for at least 2 hours before serving.
4. Store leftovers in an airtight container in the refrigerator for up to 3 days. Stir well before serving.

PREP TIP: Make this the night before or the morning before to enjoy as a refreshing treat in the afternoon on a hot summer's day.

PER SERVING: Calories: 100; Total Fat: 2g; Saturated Fat: 1g; Cholesterol: 7mg; Sodium: 94mg; Potassium: 922mg; Carbohydrates: 13g; Fiber: 2g; Sugars: 10g; Protein: 8g

Creamy Tomato Soup with Fennel

Serves 4 / Prep time: 5 minutes / Cook time: 30 minutes

This soup excites my taste buds; it's wonderful even on a warm day, and especially on a cold night. Coupled with toasted whole-grain bread or whole-grain croutons, this soup makes it onto my table as often as possible. The fennel adds a unique twist that is sure to intrigue your palate.

3 tablespoons olive oil
1½ cups chopped yellow onions
1 fennel bulb, trimmed and chopped, fronds reserved
2 carrots, chopped
1 tablespoon minced garlic

1 (28-ounce) can low-sodium tomato puree
3 cups low-sodium vegetable broth
1 tablespoon low-sodium tomato paste
1 teaspoon freshly ground black pepper
¾ cup skim milk

1. In a large heavy saucepan, heat the oil over medium heat. Add the onions, fennel, and carrots and sauté, partially covered, until the vegetables are quite tender, about 15 minutes. Add the garlic and cook for 1 minute.
2. Add the tomato puree, broth, tomato paste, and pepper and stir well. Bring the soup to a boil, reduce the heat, and simmer, uncovered, for about 15 minutes.
3. Whisk the milk into the soup. Serve garnished with the reserved fennel fronds. Store leftovers in an airtight container in the refrigerator for 3 to 4 days.

SUBSTITUTION TIP: Make this soup vegan by replacing the milk with a nondairy substitute like unsweetened almond milk or soy milk.

PER SERVING: Calories: 202; Total Fat: 11g; Saturated Fat: 2g; Cholesterol: 2mg; Sodium: 97mg; Potassium: 924mg; Carbohydrates: 23g; Fiber: 8g; Sugars: 14g; Protein: 5g

Lentil Soup

Serves 4 / Prep time: 10 minutes / Cook time: 20 minutes

Lentils are pulses, part of the legume family, the same family as beans, peas, and chickpeas. Legumes and pulses are protein- and fiber-rich plants that make a wonderful base for dishes from around the world. If you have never tried lentils, I highly recommend this soup as your introduction. They have a wonderful chewy but creamy consistency, and they lend themselves well to countless flavors, like the aromatics and vegetables in this soup.

2 teaspoons olive oil
2 cups chopped carrots
1 cup chopped onion
1 cup chopped celery
1 jalapeño, seeded and finely chopped (optional)
4 cups water

2 (15-ounce) cans low-sodium red or brown lentils, drained and rinsed
1 (15-ounce) can low-sodium tomato sauce
¼ teaspoon freshly ground black pepper
¼ cup chopped fresh cilantro

1. In a large soup pot, heat the oil over medium-high heat. Add the carrots, onion, celery, and jalapeño (if using). Cook until the vegetables begin to soften, about 6 minutes.
2. Add the water, lentils, tomato sauce, and pepper. Bring to a low boil, then reduce the heat and simmer for 15 minutes, or until the vegetables are tender.
3. Ladle into bowls, top with the cilantro, and serve. Store leftovers in an airtight container in the refrigerator for 3 to 4 days.

INGREDIENT TIP: If you don't like the spice from the jalapeño, omit it and add 1 red bell pepper, seeded and diced, instead.

PER SERVING: Calories: 276; Total Fat: 3g; Saturated Fat: 0g; Cholesterol: 0mg; Sodium: 93mg; Potassium: 1,329mg; Carbohydrates: 49g; Fiber: 17g; Sugars: 13g; Protein: 16g

ONE-POT

30 MINUTES OR LESS

DAIRY-FREE

GLUTEN-FREE

NUT-FREE

VEGAN

White Bean and Greens Soup with Sausage

Serves 6 / Prep time: 5 minutes / Cook time: 25 minutes

White beans are an excellent source of protein and are full of fiber and antioxidants. A hefty serving of super-healthy kale adds even more essential vitamins, minerals, fiber, and antioxidants. While cured meats are usually a no-go for those on low-sodium diets, this soup gets a big dose of meaty flavor from a small amount of smoked sausage. With a loaf of crusty bread and a green salad, this hearty soup makes a perfect meal for a cold evening.

2 tablespoons olive oil

1 onion, diced

2 garlic cloves, minced

2 celery stalks, sliced

2 carrots, sliced

4 ounces Spanish-style chorizo or andouille sausage, diced

1 bunch kale, stemmed and chopped

3 cups low-sodium chicken broth

1 (14.5-ounce) can low-sodium diced tomatoes

1 (15-ounce) can no-salt-added white beans, such as cannellini or great northern, drained and rinsed

1 cup water

½ teaspoon freshly ground black pepper

1. In a large stockpot, heat the oil over medium-high heat. Add the onion and garlic and cook, stirring frequently, until the onion is soft, about 5 minutes.
2. Add the celery, carrots, and sausage and cook, stirring occasionally, for 3 minutes. Stir in the kale.
3. Add the broth, tomatoes and their juices, beans, water, and pepper and bring to a boil. Reduce the heat to medium-low, cover, and simmer for about 15 minutes, until the vegetables are soft.
4. Serve hot. Store leftovers in an airtight container in the refrigerator for 3 to 4 days.

PREP TIP: Add any vegetables you prefer, like leeks or potatoes, chopped into small pieces, in step 2.

PER SERVING: Calories: 200; Total Fat: 10g; Saturated Fat: 3g; Cholesterol: 11mg; Sodium: 213mg; Potassium: 616mg; Carbohydrates: 20g; Fiber: 6g; Sugars: 4g; Protein: 8g

Parmesan-Crusted Cauliflower

Serves 4 / Prep time: 5 minutes / Cook time: 40 minutes

Cauliflower is an often overlooked vegetable, rich in important vitamins and minerals, but once you top it with a rich olive-oil-and-Parmesan crust, you will want cauliflower on your plate every night. The Parmesan adds just enough salty flavor that you won't even want to salt it at the table.

1 cauliflower head, large stems removed, cut into florets

2 tablespoons plain whole-wheat bread crumbs

1 tablespoon plus ½ teaspoon olive oil, divided

⅛ teaspoon freshly ground black pepper

1 tablespoon grated reduced-fat Parmesan cheese

1 tablespoon chopped fresh flat-leaf parsley

1. Preheat the oven to 350°F.
2. Fill a large saucepan with 1 inch of water and place a steamer basket in the pot. Put the cauliflower in the steamer basket and cover the pot. Bring the water to a boil, then reduce the heat to low and steam the cauliflower until it is crisp-tender, about 5 minutes. Transfer the cauliflower to a large bowl.
3. In a small saucepan, combine the bread crumbs, 1 tablespoon of the oil, and the pepper. Cook over medium heat, stirring, for 5 minutes.
4. Remove the pan from the heat and stir in the Parmesan and parsley. Add the bread crumb mixture to the bowl with the cauliflower and toss to coat.
5. Use the remaining ½ teaspoon oil to grease the bottom and sides of a 9-inch square baking dish. Put the cauliflower in the dish in an even layer. Roast the cauliflower until the top is golden brown, about 25 minutes.
6. Serve hot. Store leftovers in an airtight container in the refrigerator for 3 to 4 days.

PREP TIP: Make the steaming process quicker by purchasing bags of pre-cut cauliflower florets that can be steamed in the microwave.

PER SERVING: Calories: 91; Total Fat: 5g; Saturated Fat: 1g; Cholesterol: 1mg; Sodium: 83mg; Potassium: 635mg; Carbohydrates: 11g; Fiber: 4g; Sugars: 4g; Protein: 4g

Maple-Pecan Mashed Sweet Potatoes

Serves 4 / Prep time: 10 minutes / Cook time: 45 minutes

Sweet potatoes have been called a superfood, and rightfully so. They're packed with fiber, vitamins A and C, and beta-carotene, to name only a few of their nutrients. Better yet, they taste fantastic! They even smell great while they're cooking.

1 ounce raw unsalted pecans (about 20 pecan halves)
2 large sweet potatoes
2 tablespoons pure maple syrup

¼ teaspoon ground cinnamon
¼ teaspoon ground ginger
¼ teaspoon salt (optional)

1. Preheat the oven to 375°F.
2. Spread the pecans out in a single layer on a rimmed baking sheet. Roast until they are fragrant and slightly darker in color, about 5 minutes.
3. Remove the pecans from the oven and allow them to cool. Increase the oven heat to 400°F. When the pecans can be handled, chop them; you should have about ¼ cup.
4. Use a fork to poke several small holes in the skin of each potato and place them directly on the oven rack. Bake until the potatoes are fork-tender, 30 to 35 minutes. Let the potatoes cool until they can be handled.
5. In a small saucepan, combine the maple syrup, cinnamon, and ginger over medium heat. Bring to a gentle simmer. Remove the syrup from the heat and let it stand for about 5 minutes.
6. Scoop the flesh out of the cooked potatoes into a medium microwave-safe bowl. Add the salt (if using) and mash the potato flesh until smooth.
7. Mix in the syrup and the nuts and serve. Store leftovers in an airtight container in the refrigerator for up to 5 days. To warm, microwave the potatoes on high for 3 minutes before serving.

PER SERVING: Calories: 132; Total Fat: 5g; Saturated Fat: 0g; Cholesterol: 0mg; Sodium: 37mg; Potassium: 272mg; Carbohydrates: 21g; Fiber: 3g; Sugars: 9g; Protein: 2g

Roasted Balsamic Brussels Sprouts with Pecans

Serves 4 / Prep time: 5 minutes / Cook time: 20 minutes

This is a terrific recipe for those who say they don't like Brussels sprouts, as roasting them brings out their sweetness. The vinegar helps by adding a tart flavor and will make getting your daily requirement of vegetables a breeze. Substitute walnuts or almonds for the pecans, if you prefer.

20 to 25 medium Brussels sprouts, quartered
2 tablespoons olive oil

1 tablespoon balsamic vinegar
Freshly ground black pepper
¼ cup chopped unsalted toasted pecans

1. Preheat the oven to 400°F.
2. Spread the Brussels sprouts in a single layer on a baking sheet. Drizzle with the oil and vinegar, and sprinkle with pepper.
3. Roast for 15 to 20 minutes, until tender and caramelized.
4. Top with the toasted pecans and serve.

PREP TIP: If you can't find toasted pecans, you can toast the pecans during the cooking process: Sprinkle them over the Brussels sprouts about 5 minutes before the sprouts finish cooking, toss to coat in the oil in the pan, and return to the oven for the remaining cook time.

PER SERVING: Calories: 151; Total Fat: 12g; Saturated Fat: 1g; Cholesterol: 0mg; Sodium: 25mg; Potassium: 402mg; Carbohydrates: 10g; Fiber: 4g; Sugars: 3g; Protein: 4g

ONE-POT

5 INGREDIENTS OR FEWER

30 MINUTES OR LESS

DAIRY-FREE

GLUTEN-FREE

VEGAN

Brown Rice Pilaf

Serves 4 / Prep time: 5 minutes / Cook time: 60 minutes

The nutty flavor and slightly chewy texture of brown rice give this dish a bold character that's lacking in many white rice pilafs. With the addition of lemon juice, it takes on a delightful brightness. This recipe may take a long time to cook, but it's simple and mostly hands-off.

2 teaspoons olive oil
1½ cups finely chopped white or yellow onion
1¼ cups finely chopped celery stalks and leaves

1 cup brown rice
2½ cups water
2 tablespoons freshly squeezed lemon juice
¼ cup slivered raw unsalted almonds

1. In a large saucepan, heat the oil over medium heat. Add the onion and celery and cook until golden, about 5 minutes.
2. Add the rice, stir to coat, and cook for 1 minute. Add the water and lemon juice. Turn the heat up to high and bring to a boil.
3. Reduce the heat to low, cover, and simmer for 30 minutes; then start checking the rice for doneness every 5 minutes. If the pot is dry before the rice is tender, add 2 tablespoons of water. The rice should be tender and most of the liquid should be absorbed within 40 to 50 minutes.
4. Remove the rice from the heat and let it stand, covered, for 5 minutes to absorb the rest of the liquid.
5. Fluff the rice with a fork and stir in the almonds. Serve hot. Store leftovers in an airtight container in the refrigerator for 3 to 4 days.

INGREDIENT TIP: If you want even more flavor, use low-sodium chicken or vegetable broth in place of the water.

PER SERVING: Calories: 261; Total Fat: 7g; Saturated Fat: 1g; Cholesterol: 0mg; Sodium: 31mg; Potassium: 330mg; Carbohydrates: 44g; Fiber: 4g; Sugars: 4g; Protein: 6g

Aromatic Almond Couscous

Serves 4 / Prep time: 5 minutes / Cook time: 20 minutes

Although it's cooked and used like a grain, couscous is actually a pasta. It is a signature ingredient in the cuisine of North Africa, where it's served with gently spiced stews of vegetables, meat (especially lamb), and dried fruit. The cinnamon and almonds in this recipe are customary North African flavors, but feel free to experiment with other spices or nuts.

2 tablespoons olive oil
1 white or yellow onion, chopped
1½ cups low-sodium vegetable or
   chicken broth

¼ teaspoon ground cinnamon
1 cup whole-wheat instant couscous
¼ cup slivered raw unsalted almonds
¼ cup chopped fresh flat-leaf parsley

1. In a large saucepan, heat the oil over medium-low heat. Add the onion and cook until it is softened and golden, about 10 minutes.
2. Add the broth and cinnamon and bring to a boil.
3. Remove the pot from the heat and stir in the couscous. Cover the pot tightly and set it aside for 10 minutes. The couscous is done when it is tender but not mushy. If it's not soft enough, put the cover back on the pot and let stand for another 2 to 3 minutes.
4. Add the almonds and parsley and fluff the couscous with a fork. Serve warm. Store leftovers in an airtight container in the refrigerator for 3 to 4 days.

INGREDIENT TIP: If desired—and if it's within your daily sodium intake limits—add just a pinch of salt to this recipe.

PER SERVING: Calories: 274; Total Fat: 10g; Saturated Fat: 1g; Cholesterol: 0mg; Sodium: 35mg; Potassium: 183mg; Carbohydrates: 38g; Fiber: 4g; Sugars: 2g; Protein: 7g

Ginger-Lime Cilantro Noodles

Serves 4 / Prep time: 15 minutes / Cook time: 15 minutes

Cool, tangy, and light, this dish is perfect on a summer evening or alongside any spicy or rich Asian-inspired dish. The brown rice noodles have more body than the white rice version, and some people find them easier to handle. If you want to add another flavor and texture, try sesame seeds or crushed peanuts, and add just a pinch of salt.

FOR THE DRESSING

¼ cup freshly squeezed lime juice

¼ cup unseasoned rice vinegar

¼ cup chopped fresh cilantro

1 tablespoon honey

2 teaspoons toasted sesame oil

2 teaspoons grated peeled fresh ginger

2 garlic cloves, minced

1 teaspoon red pepper flakes

FOR THE SALAD

8 ounces no-salt-added Asian brown rice vermicelli

1 carrot, grated

½ seedless cucumber, peeled and grated

1 scallion (white and green parts), thinly sliced

TO MAKE THE DRESSING

1.   In a small bowl, whisk together the lime juice, rice vinegar, cilantro, honey, sesame oil, ginger, garlic, and red pepper flakes. Set aside.

TO MAKE THE SALAD

2.   Fill a large bowl two-thirds full with cold water and 1 tray of ice cubes.
3.   Cook the noodles according to the package instructions. Drain them and transfer to the ice water to cool completely. Drain well.
4.   In a large bowl, toss the noodles with the dressing, carrot, cucumber, and scallion. Serve immediately. Store leftovers in an airtight container in the refrigerator for 2 to 3 days.

PER SERVING: Calories: 216; Total Fat: 4g; Saturated Fat: 1g; Cholesterol: 0mg; Sodium: 54mg; Potassium: 256mg; Carbohydrates: 42g; Fiber: 2g; Sugars: 6g; Protein: 4g

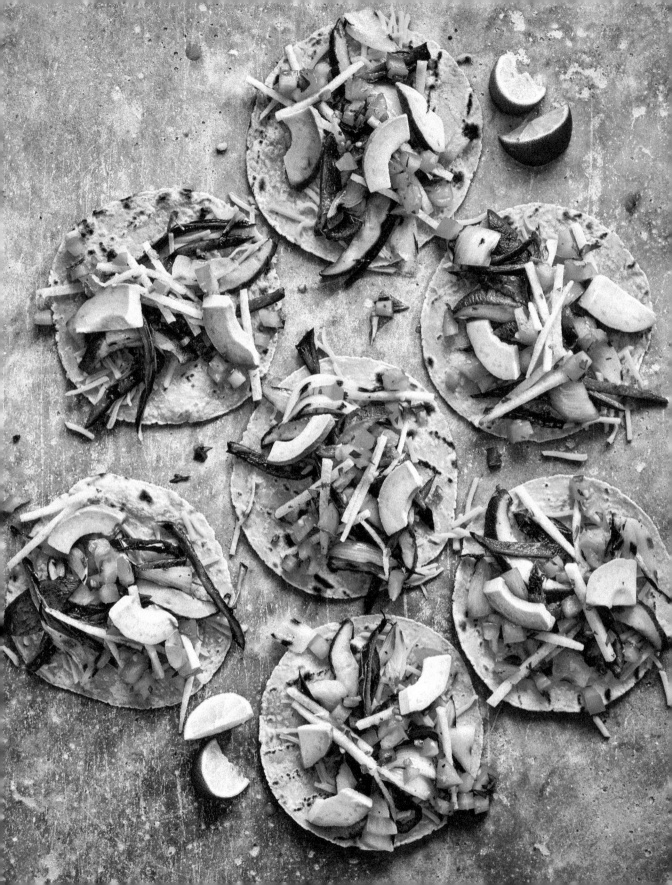

CHAPTER FOUR

Meatless Mains

Bulgur and Chickpea Salad

Serves 4 / Prep time: 5 minutes, plus 1 hour 15 minutes to chill / Cook time: 12 minutes

Bulgur is a whole grain of wheat that has been cracked, partially cooked, and dried. It comes in various grinds, from fine to extra-coarse. With all the flavor, fiber, and nutrients of unrefined wheat, bulgur has a texture that will remind you of couscous. It is a key ingredient in tabbouleh and many other Middle Eastern dishes.

FOR THE DRESSING

3 tablespoons freshly squeezed
   lemon juice
2 tablespoons olive oil
1 tablespoon minced fresh flat-leaf
   parsley

1 garlic clove, minced
½ teaspoon freshly ground black pepper

FOR THE SALAD

1 cup coarse bulgur
¾ cup canned no-salt-added chickpeas,
   drained, rinsed, and patted dry
½ cup finely chopped carrots

½ cup raisins
½ cup thinly sliced scallions (white and
   green parts)

TO MAKE THE DRESSING

1. In a small bowl, whisk together the lemon juice, oil, parsley, garlic, and pepper. Set aside.

TO MAKE THE SALAD

2. Cook the bulgur according to the package instructions, taking care that it does not become mushy, about 12 minutes. Remove it from the heat, fluff with a fork, and set aside to cool for 15 minutes.
3. In a medium bowl, mix together the cooled bulgur, chickpeas, carrots, raisins and scallions. Add the dressing and mix well.

4. Cover and chill the salad for at least 1 hour before serving. Store leftovers in an airtight container in the refrigerator for 3 to 4 days.

PREP TIP: Cook the bulgur ahead of time and keep it refrigerated to make this salad come together even quicker on a busy evening. Add ¼ teaspoon salt to the dressing if absolutely needed for flavor.

PER SERVING: Calories: 298; Total Fat: 8g; Saturated Fat: 1g; Cholesterol: 0mg; Sodium: 34mg; Potassium: 467mg; Carbohydrates: 53g; Fiber: 8g; Sugars: 14g; Protein: 8g

Southwestern Quinoa and Black Bean Salad

Serves 4 / Prep time: 15 minutes / Cook time: 15 minutes

Quinoa has pretty much everything you could want in a grain. High in fiber, quinoa is a complete protein, with all the protein components your body needs, and is a good source of calcium, magnesium, and iron. All that, and it's gluten-free, too! The small grains have a nutty flavor, similar to that of brown rice.

½ cup quinoa

2 tablespoons olive oil

1 tablespoon freshly squeezed lime juice

¼ teaspoon freshly ground black pepper

¼ teaspoon ground cumin

¼ teaspoon ground coriander

½ cup thinly sliced scallions (white and green parts)

2 tablespoons chopped fresh cilantro (optional)

1 tablespoon chopped fresh flat-leaf parsley

1 (15-ounce) can no-salt-added black beans, drained, rinsed, and patted dry

2 cups chopped tomatoes

1 red bell pepper, chopped

1 green bell pepper, chopped

2 tablespoons minced jalapeño (optional)

1. Cook the quinoa according to the package instructions; remove the pan from the heat and set it aside to cool for 15 minutes.
2. While the quinoa cooks, in a small bowl, whisk together the oil, lime juice, pepper, cumin, and coriander. Mix in the scallions, cilantro (if using), and parsley. Set aside.
3. In a large bowl, mix the beans, tomatoes, bell peppers, and jalapeño (if using). Add the cooled quinoa and stir everything together.
4. Pour the dressing over the salad and stir to coat. Serve. Store leftovers in an airtight container in the refrigerator for 3 to 4 days.

INGREDIENT TIP: You can add canned or thawed frozen corn (find a brand with no salt added) to this recipe, if desired.

PER SERVING: Calories: 260; Total Fat: 9g; Saturated Fat: 1g; Cholesterol: 0mg; Sodium: 41mg; Potassium: 723mg; Carbohydrates: 37g; Fiber: 10g; Sugars: 5g; Protein: 10g

Spinach, Chickpea, and Sweet Potato Stew

Serves 6 / Prep time: 5 minutes / Cook time: 25 minutes

This stew has just about every nutrient you could ask for, whipped up in one delicious bowl. Protein, fiber, vitamins, minerals, antioxidants, and healthy fat round out this powerhouse stew. Not to mention, the flavors are out of this world. Purchase peeled and pre-cut sweet potatoes at your grocery store to make this even easier to prep.

2 tablespoons canola oil
1 yellow onion, chopped
4 garlic cloves, minced
1 tablespoon grated peeled fresh ginger
Grated zest and juice of 1 lemon, divided
¼ teaspoon red pepper flakes
2 tablespoons low-sodium
  tomato paste

1 (15-ounce) can no-salt-added
  chickpeas, drained and rinsed
2 sweet potatoes, peeled and diced
1 (13.5-ounce) can lite coconut milk
1 teaspoon ground ginger
1 pound baby spinach
¼ cup chopped fresh cilantro, for garnish
  (optional)

1. In a large stockpot, heat the oil over medium-high heat. Add the onion and cook, stirring occasionally, until softened and beginning to brown, about 5 minutes.
2. Stir in the garlic, ginger, lemon zest, and red pepper flakes and cook, stirring frequently, for about 3 minutes. Stir in the tomato paste and cook for 1 minute, then add the chickpeas and sweet potatoes.
3. Raise the heat to high and cook for about 3 minutes. Add the coconut milk and ginger, stir to mix, and heat until simmering. Reduce the heat to low and cook until the sweet potatoes are tender, about 15 minutes.
4. Add the spinach by the handful, letting each handful wilt before adding another, and cook for a few minutes to ensure that the spinach is fully cooked and warmed through. Stir in the lemon juice.
5. Serve hot, garnished with the cilantro, if desired. Store leftovers in an airtight container in the refrigerator for 3 to 4 days.

PER SERVING: Calories: 274; Total Fat: 16g; Saturated Fat: 9g; Cholesterol: 0mg; Sodium: 97mg; Potassium: 896mg; Carbohydrates: 28g; Fiber: 7g; Sugars: 6g; Protein: 8g

Curried Chickpea Mediterranean Wrap

Serves 2 / Prep time: 15 minutes

Chickpeas are a plant-based food loaded with protein and fiber, and they make a fantastic sandwich filling. Research has shown that including these tasty legumes in your meals can reduce your consumption of processed foods and keep you satisfied longer.

1 (15-ounce) can no-salt-added chickpeas, drained and rinsed
½ cup green grapes, halved
1 celery stalk, finely chopped
¼ red onion, finely chopped
2 tablespoons low-fat plain yogurt

2 tablespoons chopped raw unsalted cashews
1 teaspoon curry powder
2 (8-inch) whole-wheat tortillas
1 cup alfalfa sprouts

1. Put the chickpeas in a medium bowl and mash until chunky.
2. Add the grapes, celery, onion, yogurt, cashews, and curry powder and stir until the mixture is thoroughly combined.
3. Lay out the tortillas on a clean work surface. Spread with the filling, dividing it evenly among the tortillas.
4. Top with the sprouts and fold the tortillas to form tight pockets. Serve.

SUBSTITUTION TIP: Wrap the chickpea filling in butter lettuce leaves to lower the calories and carb count in this recipe.

PER SERVING: Calories: 430; Total Fat: 12g; Saturated Fat: 3g; Cholesterol: 1mg; Sodium: 249mg; Potassium: 719mg; Carbohydrates: 66g; Fiber: 15g; Sugars: 15g; Protein: 18g

Whole-Wheat Mu Shu Vegetable-Inspired Wraps

Serves 4 / Prep time: 5 minutes / Cook time: 10 minutes

Full of protein, whole grains, and vegetables, these warm and crunchy vegetarian wraps are on your table in just 15 minutes, making them a great option for a busy-night dinner or work-from-home lunch. They also are delicious chilled, or can be reheated for a grab-and-go lunch.

3 teaspoons toasted sesame oil, divided
4 large eggs, lightly beaten
2 teaspoons minced peeled fresh ginger
2 garlic cloves, minced
1 (12-ounce) bag shredded coleslaw mix
   or broccoli slaw
2 cups bean sprouts

1 bunch scallions (white and green parts),
   sliced, divided
1 tablespoon low-sodium soy sauce
1 tablespoon unseasoned rice vinegar
2 tablespoons hoisin sauce
4 whole-wheat tortillas

1. In a large sauté pan or skillet, heat 1 teaspoon of the oil over medium heat. Add the eggs and cook, stirring, for about 3 minutes, until just set. Transfer the eggs to a plate.
2. In the same skillet, heat the remaining 2 teaspoons oil over medium heat. Add the ginger and garlic and cook for 1 minute.
3. Stir in the coleslaw mix, bean sprouts, half the scallions, the soy sauce, and the vinegar. Cover and cook for about 3 minutes, until the vegetables are tender. Return the cooked eggs to the pan, add the hoisin sauce, and cook, stirring, for about 2 minutes. Remove from the heat and add the remaining scallions.
4. Warm the tortillas according to the package instructions. Place the tortillas on serving plates and divide the vegetable mixture among them. Roll up each tortilla with the veggies tightly inside and serve immediately.
5. To store leftovers, store the egg-vegetable mixture in an airtight container in the refrigerator for up to 3 days and heat in the microwave before wrapping in tortillas and serving.

PER SERVING: Calories: 290; Total Fat: 13g; Saturated Fat: 4g; Cholesterol: 186mg; Sodium: 521mg; Potassium: 586mg; Carbohydrates: 30g; Fiber: 8g; Sugars: 5g; Protein: 16g

Grilled Mushroom Tacos with Fresh Salsa

Serves 4 / Prep time: 10 minutes / Cook time: 15 minutes

Mushrooms are a wonderful nutrient-dense food that have a unique meaty texture, often finding their place as meat substitutes in vegetarian cooking. These tacos are a flavor explosion, sure to please even the pickiest of palates. If you don't have a grill, use the broil setting on the oven to roast the veggies. Roast on a baking sheet for 5 to 10 minutes on each side or until tender.

FOR THE SALSA

3 plum tomatoes, seeded and chopped
½ cup thinly sliced jicama
1 serrano chile, minced

2 tablespoons chopped fresh cilantro
2 tablespoons freshly squeezed lime juice
⅛ teaspoon red pepper flakes

FOR THE TACOS

4 portobello mushroom caps, gills
    scraped out and discarded
4 (¼-inch-thick) slices onion
1 whole poblano chile
1 tablespoon olive oil
3 garlic cloves, thinly sliced

½ teaspoon ground cumin
8 (6-inch) corn tortillas
1 avocado, pitted and sliced
1 cup shredded reduced-fat
    Cheddar cheese

TO MAKE THE SALSA

1. In a small bowl, combine the tomatoes, jicama, serrano, cilantro, lime juice, and red pepper flakes, and mix well. Set aside.

TO MAKE THE TACOS

2. Heat a grill to medium-hgh heat.
3. Grill the mushrooms, onion, and poblano until tender, about 5 minutes per side. Seed the poblano, remove the stem, and cut it into thin strips. Cut the mushrooms into thin strips. Chop the onion. In a medium bowl, mix the grilled vegetables together.
4. In a large nonstick skillet, heat the oil over medium-high heat. Add the garlic and cook, stirring, for 1 minute. Add the vegetable mixture and the cumin and cook until thoroughly heated, about 2 minutes.
5. Heat the tortillas according to the package instructions. For each serving, place two tortillas on a plate. Top each tortilla with some of the mushroom mixture, the salsa, and a few slices of avocado. Top each taco with about 2 tablespoons of the cheese. Serve immediately. Store leftover mushroom mixture and toppings in separate airtight containers in the refrigerator for 1 to 2 days.

PER SERVING: Calories: 330; Total Fat: 15g; Saturated Fat: 3g; Cholesterol: 6mg; Sodium: 269mg; Potassium: 871mg; Carbohydrates: 41g; Fiber: 9g; Sugars: 6g; Protein: 14g

Black-Eyed Pea Burgers

Serves 4 / Prep time: 10 minutes / Cook time: 15 minutes

Mushrooms are moist, tender, and loaded with umami, the savory basic taste intrinsic to certain foods. The addition of umami-rich foods lends a pleasant meatiness to vegetarian and nonvegetarian dishes alike. These rich, tasty burgers are loaded with micronutrients and iron. Try them without bread—you may find them filling enough on their own.

5 tablespoons grapeseed or olive oil, divided

4 ounces cremini mushrooms, stemmed and sliced

¼ teaspoon dried thyme

½ chopped red onion, plus more for serving

2 garlic cloves, minced

1 (15-ounce) can no-salt-added black-eyed peas, drained and rinsed

2 tablespoons minced fresh basil or flat-leaf parsley

½ teaspoon tamari

4 large butter lettuce leaves

1 avocado, pitted and sliced

1. In a large sauté pan, heat 3 tablespoons of the oil over medium heat until shimmering. Add the mushrooms and thyme and cook, stirring occasionally, until the mushrooms are browned, 2 to 3 minutes. Add the onion and garlic and cook until fragrant and softened, about 2 minutes. Remove from the heat.

2. Place the black-eyed peas in a large bowl and mash with the back of a spoon or a potato masher, leaving a few of the peas intact. Add the mushroom mixture, basil, and tamari and mix until combined. Form the mixture into four patties.

3. In the same sauté pan, heat the remaining 2 tablespoons oil over medium-high heat until shimmering. Add the patties and fry until browned, 5 to 6 minutes per side.

4. Serve on lettuce leaves with additional red onion and avocado. Store leftover burgers in an airtight container in the refrigerator for 3 to 4 days.

SUBSTITUTION TIP: If you prefer black beans to black-eyed peas, feel free to swap those in.

PER SERVING: Calories: 340; Total Fat: 25g; Saturated Fat: 4g; Cholesterol: 0mg; Sodium: 53mg; Potassium: 667mg; Carbohydrates: 25g; Fiber: 10g; Sugars: 3g; Protein: 8g

Vegetarian Kebabs

Serves 4 / Prep time: 15 minutes, plus 30 minutes to marinate / Cook time: 10 minutes

If you have a grill, make these delicious kebabs over a medium fire. You can use any combination of vegetables on the skewer, such as baby portobello mushrooms, red or yellow bell peppers, sweet potato chunks, or eggplant. Get a nice assortment of colors so you get a broad range of phytonutrients on your plate. Serve with a side of rice or quinoa, if desired.

¼ cup olive oil

2 tablespoons balsamic vinegar

1 teaspoon minced garlic

½ teaspoon chopped fresh thyme

½ teaspoon chopped fresh oregano

Freshly ground black pepper

2 small zucchini, cut into 16 chunks total

2 small white or red onions, cut into quarters

16 cherry tomatoes

16 medium button mushrooms

2 cups broccoli florets

2 red, yellow, or green bell peppers, cut into 8 slices each

1. In a large zip-top plastic bag, combine the oil, vinegar, garlic, thyme, oregano, and black pepper. Add the zucchini, onions, tomatoes, mushrooms, broccoli, and bell peppers, zip closed, and shake well to coat.
2. Place in the refrigerator for at least 30 minutes. Meanwhile, if using wooden skewers, soak 8 of them in water.
3. Preheat the broiler with an oven rack about 6 inches from the broiler.
4. Take the vegetables out of fridge and thread them onto skewers, placing two zucchini pieces, one piece of onion, two tomatoes, two mushrooms, two broccoli florets, and two pieces of bell pepper on each skewer. Reserve the remaining marinade.
5. Place the skewers on a baking sheet or oven grill rack and broil, turning once and basting with the reserved marinade, until the vegetables are tender, about 10 minutes. Serve hot. Store leftovers in an airtight container in the refrigerator for 3 to 4 days.

PER SERVING: Calories: 221; Total Fat: 14g; Saturated Fat: 2g; Cholesterol: 0mg; Sodium: 32mg; Potassium: 950mg; Carbohydrates: 21g; Fiber: 5g; Sugars: 8g; Protein: 6g

Mushroom-Stuffed Zucchini

Serves 2 / Prep time: 5 minutes / Cook time: 50 minutes

Fresh zucchini with mushrooms seasoned with garlic, olive oil, parsley, herbs, and spices hardly seems like "healthy" food. These mushroom-stuffed zucchini boats make an easy and impressive dish that is low in calories but still filling. For added flavor, use low-sodium chicken or vegetable broth instead of water and top with a sprinkle of reduced-fat Parmesan cheese.

2 medium zucchini, halved lengthwise

2 tablespoons olive oil

2 cups finely chopped button mushrooms

2 garlic cloves, finely chopped

1 tablespoon finely chopped fresh flat-leaf parsley

1 tablespoon Italian seasoning

Freshly ground black pepper

2 tablespoons water

1. Preheat the oven to 350°F.
2. Scoop out the insides of the zucchini halves and place the halves cut-side up inside a casserole dish. Set aside.
3. In a large skillet, heat the oil over medium heat. Add the mushrooms and cook until tender, about 4 minutes.
4. Add the garlic and cook for 2 minutes more.
5. Add the parsley and Italian seasoning and season with pepper. Stir and remove from the heat. Stuff each zucchini with the mushroom mixture.
6. Drizzle the water into the bottom of the dish. Cover with foil and bake for 30 to 40 minutes, until the zucchini are tender.
7. Serve immediately. Store leftovers in an airtight container in the refrigerator for 3 to 4 days.

PER SERVING: Calories: 175; Total Fat: 14g; Saturated Fat: 2g; Cholesterol: 0mg; Sodium: 21mg; Potassium: 763mg; Carbohydrates: 10g; Fiber: 3g; Sugars: 6g; Protein: 5g

Ratatouille Pasta

Serves 6 / Prep time: 10 minutes / Cook time: 25 minutes

Eating plenty of vegetables is a great strategy for general good health and goes a long way toward meeting DASH goals. This Mediterranean-inspired pasta dish is bursting with flavor and nutritious, colorful produce. You can also serve the ratatouille with brown rice instead of pasta or eat it plain as a stew.

DAIRY-FREE

NUT-FREE

VEGAN

12 ounces multigrain spaghetti
1 tablespoon olive oil
1 large sweet onion, chopped
1 tablespoon minced garlic
1 small eggplant, cut into ½-inch cubes
2 small green zucchini, diced

1 red bell pepper, diced
2 large tomatoes, diced
½ teaspoon freshly ground black pepper
Pinch red pepper flakes
2 tablespoons chopped fresh basil

1. Cook the pasta according to the package instructions. Drain and set aside.
2. While the pasta cooks, in a large skillet, heat the oil over medium-high heat. Add the onion and garlic and sauté until tender, about 4 minutes.
3. Add the eggplant, zucchini, and bell pepper. Sauté until softened, about 10 minutes.
4. Add the tomato, black pepper, and red pepper flakes. Cook, stirring occasionally, until the vegetables are tender and the liquid reduces to a sauce texture, about 7 minutes.
5. Stir in the basil and cooked pasta, and cook, stirring occasionally, until the pasta is warmed through, about 4 minutes. Serve hot. Store leftovers in an airtight container in the refrigerator for 3 to 4 days.

PREP TIP: Purchase pre-cut vegetables to make this recipe even quicker to prepare.

PER SERVING: Calories: 284; Total Fat: 4g; Saturated Fat: 1g; Cholesterol: 0mg; Sodium: 24mg; Potassium: 693mg; Carbohydrates: 57g; Fiber: 9g; Sugars: 9g; Protein: 11g

Pasta Caprese

Serves 6 / Prep time: 10 minutes, plus 1 hour to rest / Cook time: 10 minutes

This dish is essentially a caprese salad tossed with pasta. The mini moz-zarella balls add richness, and the tomato and basil bring bright color and nutrients. Use whole-wheat pasta if you're watching your sodium intake. The difference between whole-wheat pasta and white-flour pasta is a whopping 136 mg of sodium. The tiny balls of marinated mozzarella used here are called bocconcini, and they also make great appetizers and snacks.

1 pound bocconcini (mozzarella balls),
  drained and halved
1 pound small tomatoes, sliced
¾ cup olive oil

Leaves from 1 large bunch basil
Freshly ground black pepper
12 ounces whole-wheat spaghetti

1. In a large bowl, combine the bocconcini, tomatoes, oil, and basil. Toss to com-bine and season with pepper to taste. Allow the mixture to rest for at least 1 hour to let the cheese soften and flavors develop.
2. Cook the spaghetti according to the package instructions. Drain and rinse with cold water until the pasta is cool.
3. Add the pasta and basil to the bocconcini mixture and toss well. Serve. Store leftovers in an airtight container in the refrigerator for 2 to 3 days.

INGREDIENT TIP: Add a drizzle of balsamic vinegar or balsamic reduction for an even more flavorful take on this recipe. For a lower sodium content, reduce the amount of mozzarella called for in this recipe.

PER SERVING: Calories: 677; Total Fat: 45g; Saturated Fat: 13g; Cholesterol: 60mg; Sodium: 483mg; Potassium: 371mg; Carbohydrates: 47g; Fiber: 6g; Sugars: 3g; Protein: 26g

Spicy Broccoli and Noodles

Serves 4 / Prep time: 10 minutes / Cook time: 20 minutes

Stir-frying is one of the healthier techniques for cooking. It uses minimal fat, and the food is usually not drenched in sodium-laced sauces. You can add a teaspoon of low-sodium soy sauce to this dish without going outside of DASH recommendations, but these noodles are delicious without it.

1 (8-ounce) package rice noodles

1 tablespoon toasted sesame oil

1 tablespoon minced garlic

1 tablespoon grated peeled fresh ginger

2 scallions (white and green parts), thinly sliced, divided

2 medium carrots, thinly sliced into disks

1 cup small broccoli florets

1 cup sliced mushrooms

1 cup halved snow peas, strings removed

1 cup bean sprouts

1 cup lightly packed shredded spinach

Red pepper flakes

¼ cup chopped roasted unsalted almonds

1. In a large saucepan, cook the rice noodles according to the package instructions. Drain and set aside.
2. In the same pan, heat the oil over medium-high heat. Add the garlic and ginger and sauté until softened, about 3 minutes.
3. Add the scallions, reserving 2 tablespoons for garnish, and sauté until softened, about 1 minute. Add the carrots and broccoli and stir-fry until the vegetables are crisp-tender, about 4 minutes.
4. Add the mushrooms and snow peas and stir-fry for about 2 minutes. Stir in the bean sprouts and spinach and stir-fry until the spinach is wilted, about 2 minutes or less.
5. Remove the pan from the heat and stir in the red pepper flakes. Add the rice noodles and toss with the vegetables until well combined.
6. Serve hot, topped with the almonds and reserved scallions. Store leftovers in an airtight container in the refrigerator for 1 to 2 days.

PREP TIP: Purchase a package of pre-cut stir-fry vegetables to make this recipe even quicker.

PER SERVING: Calories: 328; Total Fat: 8g; Saturated Fat: 1g; Cholesterol: 0mg; Sodium: 144mg; Potassium: 486mg; Carbohydrates: 57g; Fiber: 5g; Sugars: 3g; Protein: 9g

ONE-POT

30 MINUTES OR LESS

DAIRY-FREE

GLUTEN-FREE

VEGAN

Cold Soba Noodles with Peanut Sauce

Serves 4 / Prep time: 10 minutes / Cook time: 20 minutes

Soba noodles are packed with thiamine, a B vitamin that aids the body in the breakdown of carbohydrates. A word of caution: The sodium levels in soba noodles vary wildly, so be sure to check the label. For the peanut sauce, buy creamy natural peanut butter with no sugar or salt added and the oil separated out.

FOR THE NOODLES

1 (8-ounce) package 100% organic buckwheat soba noodles
Nonstick cooking spray
1 red bell pepper, sliced into thin strips
2 cups small broccoli florets
1 cup fresh cilantro leaves, plus 4 cilantro sprigs for garnish

1 small bunch scallions (white and green parts), thinly sliced
Chopped raw unsalted peanuts, for garnish

FOR THE PEANUT SAUCE

1 cup creamy unsalted natural peanut butter
½ cup canned lite coconut milk

1 tablespoon freshly squeezed lime juice, plus more for serving

TO MAKE THE NOODLES

1. Cook the noodles according to the package instructions. Drain in a colander and run cold water over them to stop the cooking process. Cover with a damp dish towel and set aside.

2. Spray a large sauté pan or skillet with cooking spray and place over medium-high heat. When the pan is hot, add the bell pepper and sauté until soft, about 5 minutes. Transfer to a bowl and set aside. Spray the pan again and sauté the broccoli just until the florets are bright green but still firm, 3 to 5 minutes. Add to the bell pepper.

3. In a large bowl, combine the cooled noodles and cooked vegetables and toss well. Stir in the cilantro and scallions.

TO MAKE THE PEANUT SAUCE

4. Combine the peanut butter, coconut milk, and lime juice in a blender or food processor and blend until smooth.
5. Pour the sauce over the noodles and toss well to combine. Divide the noodles among four bowls, sprinkle a little lime juice over the top, garnish with the peanuts and cilantro sprigs, and serve. Store leftovers in an airtight container in the refrigerator for 2 to 3 days.

INGREDIENT TIP: Add shredded cooked chicken or your favorite protein to this recipe, if desired.

PER SERVING: Calories: 661; Total Fat: 40g; Saturated Fat: 10g; Cholesterol: 0mg; Sodium: 34mg; Potassium: 756mg; Carbohydrates: 65g; Fiber: 9g; Sugars: 9g; Protein: 26g

Quinoa with Vegetables and Toasted Pecans

Serves 4 / Prep time: 5 minutes / Cook time: 25 minutes

If quinoa was the fuel that built the Aztec civilization, imagine what it can do for you. Fresh vegetables and herbs weave color throughout this dish, and a simple vinaigrette holds it together. Quinoa is perfect for experimenting with: Use this recipe as a starting point and then modify it to try different vegetables, nuts, and dried fruits in whatever combinations please you.

FOR THE QUINOA

2 tablespoons olive oil

2 cups quinoa, rinsed and drained well

3 cups low-sodium vegetable broth

½ cup whole raw unsalted pecans

1 cup halved cherry tomatoes

½ cup shredded carrot

½ cup finely diced zucchini

¼ cup dried currants

FOR THE VINAIGRETTE

¼ cup freshly squeezed lemon juice

2 tablespoons minced shallot

Freshly ground black pepper

¾ cup olive or walnut oil

TO MAKE THE QUINOA

1. In a large sauté pan or skillet, heat the oil over medium-high heat. Add the quinoa and toast, stirring frequently, for 2 to 3 minutes. Be sure to watch closely, as it burns quickly.
2. In a large pot, bring the broth to a boil and add the toasted quinoa. Simmer for 15 to 17 minutes. Drain and transfer to a large bowl.
3. Meanwhile, in a small skillet pan, toast the pecans over medium-high heat. Stir frequently to keep them from scorching and remove immediately from the heat once crisp, as they will burn quickly.
4. Add the pecans, tomatoes, carrot, zucchini, and currants to the quinoa and mix thoroughly.

TO MAKE THE VINAIGRETTE

5. In a small bowl, whisk together the lemon juice and shallot. Add pepper to taste. Drizzle the oil into the mixture in a thin stream, whisking constantly.

6. Pour the vinaigrette over the quinoa and vegetables and toss thoroughly. Serve immediately.

SERVING TIP: This dish will keep in the refrigerator for a day or two, developing even more flavor. Bring it to room temperature, drizzle on a little more oil to rehydrate, and serve.

PER SERVING: Calories: 877; Total Fat: 63g; Saturated Fat: 6g; Cholesterol: 0mg; Sodium: 24mg; Potassium: 835mg; Carbohydrates: 68g; Fiber: 9g; Sugars: 10g; Protein: 14g

Cheesy Vegetarian Rice Casserole

Serves 4 / Prep time: 10 minutes / Cook time: 50 minutes

Casseroles are one of my favorite dishes to whip up, because they are a one-pan meal that are essentially bake-and-eat, with minimal prep and monitoring. Even better, casseroles (like soups) taste more delicious as leftovers, so this recipe makes a great freezer meal to pull out on a busy night or for leftovers throughout the week.

2 cups chopped broccoli

1 cup chopped spinach

1 cup chopped cauliflower

½ cup diced carrot

½ cup diced red bell pepper

1 teaspoon paprika

¼ teaspoon freshly ground black pepper

¾ cup medium-grain brown rice

½ cup shredded reduced-fat Swiss cheese

1 cup plain unsweetened almond milk

½ cup low-fat plain yogurt

1. Preheat the oven to 375°F.
2. In a 9-by-13-inch glass baking dish, combine the broccoli, spinach, cauliflower, carrot, and bell pepper. Add the paprika and black pepper and toss well with tongs to distribute evenly. Add the rice and cheese and toss again to combine.
3. In a small bowl, mix together the almond milk and yogurt, and pour the mixture over the casserole. Cover with foil and bake for 50 minutes, or until the rice is tender.
4. Serve hot. Store leftovers in an airtight container in the refrigerator for 3 to 4 days.

PREP TIP: Purchase pre-chopped veggies to make this recipe even quicker and more hands-off.

PER SERVING: Calories: 229; Total Fat: 4g; Saturated Fat: 1g; Cholesterol: 7mg; Sodium: 111mg; Potassium: 619mg; Carbohydrates: 38g; Fiber: 4g; Sugars: 6g; Protein: 12g

Roasted Vegetable Pizza

Serves 4 / Prep time: 10 minutes / Cook time: 30 minutes

Pizza is a crowd-pleasing favorite that is just as delicious without meat. You will not miss the pepperoni or Italian sausage on this pie thanks to the meaty mushrooms and eggplant and the vibrant veggie flavors.

½ bunch asparagus, cut into 3-inch
  pieces
½ small red onion, sliced into half rounds
½ small red bell pepper, sliced
½ cup sliced mushrooms
½ small eggplant, cut into quarter rounds

2 tablespoons olive oil
¼ cup low-sodium pizza sauce
1 pre-made whole-wheat pizza crust
½ cup grated low-fat mozzarella cheese
1 teaspoon Italian herb blend

1. Preheat the oven to 400°F. Line a baking sheet with foil.
2. Combine the asparagus, onion, bell pepper, mushrooms, and eggplant on the prepared baking sheet. Drizzle with oil and toss until evenly coated.
3. Arrange in a single layer on the baking sheet and roast for 15 to 20 minutes, until tender. Remove from the oven.
4. Spread the sauce over the crust in a thin layer. Arrange the vegetables on top and sprinkle evenly with the mozzarella and herb blend.
5. Place the pizza on the same baking sheet and bake for 5 to 10 minutes, until the cheese is melted and the crust is crisp. Serve hot. Store leftovers in an airtight container in the refrigerator for 3 to 4 days.

INGREDIENT TIP: Make your own salt-free Italian herb blend using dried oregano, dried marjoram, dried thyme, dried basil, dried rosemary, and dried sage.

PER SERVING: Calories: 199; Total Fat: 8g; Saturated Fat: 1g; Cholesterol: 3mg; Sodium: 252mg; Potassium: 380mg; Carbohydrates: 26g; Fiber: 6g; Sugars: 5g; Protein: 9g

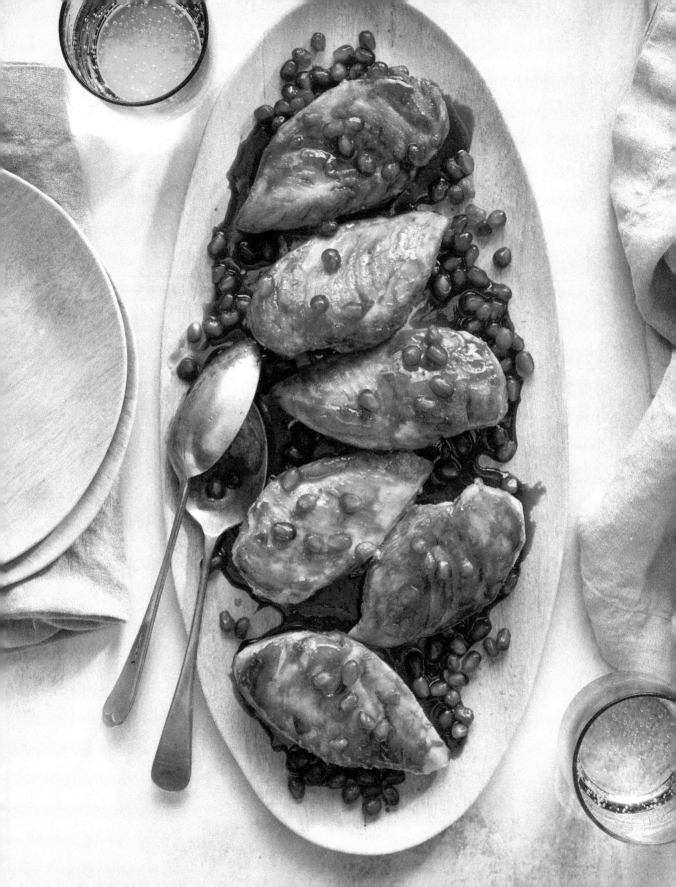

CHAPTER FIVE

Seafood and Poultry Mains

Mini Crab Cakes on Baby Greens

Serves 6 / Prep time: 15 minutes / Cook time: 10 minutes

Crab cakes are a crowd favorite but are often very high in sodium. Here we decrease the salt and add red bell pepper, scallions, and parsley to turn these crab cakes into the perfect hit of protein and vitamin C. Pile two cakes atop a simple green salad rich in iron, vitamin A, and fiber, and lunch or dinner is served. Real mayonnaise is called for because the calorie difference between it and light mayo is minimal, but there's more sodium in reduced-fat versions.

FOR THE SALAD

1 (5-ounce) package spring greens mix

2 to 3 tablespoons olive oil

2 tablespoons balsamic vinegar

Freshly ground black pepper

FOR THE CRAB CAKES

½ cup whole-wheat panko bread crumbs

1 large egg, beaten

2 to 3 tablespoons real mayonnaise

2 scallions (white and green parts), finely chopped

3 tablespoons finely chopped red bell pepper

1 teaspoon ground cayenne pepper

12 ounces lump crabmeat

2 tablespoons skim milk

2 tablespoons olive oil

2 tablespoons freshly squeezed lemon juice

2 tablespoons finely chopped fresh flat-leaf parsley leaves

TO MAKE THE SALAD

1. In a large bowl, drizzle the greens with oil, tossing until the leaves are coated.
2. Drizzle the greens with the balsamic vinegar, making sure each leaf is lightly dressed.
3. Season with pepper to taste. Divide the salad among plates.

TO MAKE THE CRAB CAKES

4. In a large bowl, combine the bread crumbs, egg, mayonnaise, scallions, bell pepper, and cayenne. Mix thoroughly.
5. Break apart and pick through the crabmeat, discarding any shell pieces. Gently fold the milk into the crabmeat. Stir into the egg mixture to incorporate well.
6. Take a heaping tablespoon of the crab mixture, pat it into a small patty, and set it on a cutting board or baking sheet. Repeat with the remaining crab mixture; you should have eight to ten patties.
7. In a large sauté pan or skillet, heat the oil over medium-high heat. Add the crab cakes and cook for about 3 minutes on each side. Watch closely and adjust the cooking time as needed to avoid burning. Drain the crab cakes on paper towels.
8. Place two warm crab cakes in the center of each plate. Squirt a little lemon on each cake, sprinkle with parsley, and serve immediately. Store leftover crab cakes and salad greens in separate airtight containers in the refrigerator for 1 to 2 days.

SUBSTITUTION TIP: To make this recipe gluten-free, substitute low-sodium gluten-free panko bread crumbs.

PER SERVING: Calories: 204; Total Fat: 14g; Saturated Fat: 2g; Cholesterol: 67mg; Sodium: 228mg; Potassium: 338mg; Carbohydrates: 7g; Fiber: 1g; Sugars: 2g; Protein: 12g

Spicy Grilled Prawn Skewers and Cucumber-Cashew Salad

Serves 4 / Prep time: 10 minutes / Cook time: 6 minutes

Prawns are a wonderful quick-cooking lean protein that takes on the flavors you choose. The spicy rub in this recipe pairs perfectly with the refreshing cucumber-cashew salad. This recipe provides a delightful mixture of textures, temperatures, and flavors sure to excite your palate. Use metal skewers if you have them to eliminate soaking time.

FOR THE CUCUMBER SALAD

2 cucumbers, peeled, seeded, and diced
½ cup coarsely chopped roasted unsalted cashews
¼ cup chopped fresh flat-leaf parsley

2 scallions (white and green parts), thinly sliced
2 tablespoons olive oil
1 tablespoon freshly squeezed lemon juice

FOR THE PRAWN SKEWERS

1 serrano chile, seeded and finely minced
1 tablespoon olive oil
1 teaspoon ground cumin

1 teaspoon chili powder
1½ pounds large or jumbo shrimp, thawed (if frozen), peeled, and deveined

TO MAKE THE SALAD

1. In a large bowl, toss the cucumbers, cashews, parsley, scallions, oil, and lemon juice.
2. Refrigerate and allow to marinate before serving.

TO MAKE THE PRAWNS

3. Soak four wooden skewers in water. Heat a grill to medium-high.
4. In a large bowl, combine the serrano chile, oil, cumin, and chili powder. Add the prawns to the bowl and toss to coat with the spice mixture.
5. Thread the prawns onto the skewers. Grill the prawns for about 3 minutes per side, until they are pink and cooked through. Serve atop the cucumber salad.
6. Store leftovers in an airtight container in the refrigerator for up to 3 days.

PER SERVING: Calories: 473; Total Fat: 28g; Saturated Fat: 5g; Cholesterol: 274mg; Sodium: 234mg; Potassium: 991mg; Carbohydrates: 19g; Fiber: 3g; Sugars: 5g; Protein: 42g

Noodle Salad with Shrimp and Cucumber

Serves 4 / Prep time: 10 minutes / Cook time: 15 minutes

In this recipe, shrimp is gently simmered in spiced oil and vinegar and then paired with cool cucumber. In cooking, always think opposites—spicy and mild, sweet and sour, smooth and crunchy—to create interesting textures and flavors. Serve this at room temperature or chill for 30 to 60 minutes before serving.

2 cups whole-wheat pasta, such as penne or fusilli
¼ cup white wine vinegar
2 tablespoons dried oregano
2 garlic cloves, finely chopped

¼ cup olive oil
1 pound shrimp, peeled and deveined
1 cucumber, peeled, seeded, quartered lengthwise, and thinly sliced

1. Cook the pasta until al dente according to the package instructions. Do not overcook. Drain and run cold water over the pasta to stop the cooking. Drain again, and then transfer to a large bowl.
2. In a small bowl, stir together the vinegar, oregano, and garlic. While whisking constantly, slowly drizzle in the oil. Pour into a small skillet and place over medium heat. Add the shrimp to the hot oil mixture and cook until they turn pink, about 3 minutes.
3. Add the shrimp and the oil mixture to the pasta, stir in the cucumber, and toss the salad thoroughly to coat. Serve. Store leftovers in an airtight container in the refrigerator for up to 3 days.

PER SERVING: Calories: 414; Total Fat: 15g; Saturated Fat: 2g; Cholesterol: 183mg; Sodium: 142mg; Potassium: 511mg; Carbohydrates: 42g; Fiber: 5g; Sugars: 1g; Protein: 31g

Ginger-Spiced Haddock Fillets

Serves 4 / Prep time: 5 minutes, plus 1 hour to marinate / Cook time: 5 minutes

Rich in omega-3 fatty acids, haddock is a firm, moist fish that absorbs seasoning and flavors well. You can substitute cod or flounder if haddock isn't available. Serve this over rice and steamed vegetables, drizzling the pan sauce over everything for a touch of decadence.

¼ cup orange juice

2 tablespoons olive oil, divided

2 teaspoons grated peeled fresh ginger

2 teaspoons honey

1 teaspoon Dijon mustard

1 tablespoon unseasoned rice vinegar

2 teaspoons low-sodium soy sauce

4 (6-ounce) haddock fillets

1 cup chopped scallions (white and green parts)

10 cherry tomatoes, halved

1. In a zip-top bag, combine the orange juice, 1 tablespoon of the oil, the ginger, honey, mustard, vinegar, and soy sauce. Add the fish fillets, seal the bag, and marinate in the refrigerator for 1 hour.
2. Heat a large heavy skillet over medium-high heat. Add the remaining 1 tablespoon oil and heat for 1 minute. Add the fish fillets, reserving the marinade, then arrange the scallions and tomatoes around the edges of the pan. Cook for 1 minute.
3. Turn the fish over, reduce the heat to low, and pour the marinade over the fish. Cover and cook for 3 minutes, or until cooked through. Serve. Store leftovers in an airtight container in the refrigerator for up to 3 days.

PER SERVING: Calories: 222; Total Fat: 8g; Saturated Fat: 1g; Cholesterol: 92mg; Sodium: 464mg; Potassium: 705mg; Total Carbohydrate: 8g; Fiber: 1g; Sugars: 6g; Protein: 29g

Citrus-Kissed Flounder in Foil

Serves 4 / Prep time: 10 minutes / Cook time: 20 minutes

This is a wonderful way to cook delicious fish with no muss and no fuss. The orange and lime add just the right amount of freshness, and there's no pan to wash when you're done. Plus, you'll also get a healthful dose of potassium.

4 (6-ounce) flounder fillets
1 teaspoon olive oil
½ teaspoon freshly ground black pepper
8 thin orange slices
8 thin lime slices

4 rosemary sprigs
Juice of 1 orange
Juice of 1 small lime
½ cup dry white wine

1. Preheat the oven to 400°F. Cut four 12-inch lengths of foil and lay them out on a clean work surface or counter.
2. Rub each fish fillet with oil and season both sides with pepper. Place each fillet on one sheet of foil. Alternate slices of orange and lime on each fillet, allocating two slices of each fruit per fillet.
3. Lay the rosemary sprigs on top of the fruit slices, and squeeze both orange and lime juice over each fillet. Pour one-quarter of the wine over the first fillet, quickly fold the edges of the foil up at the ends, and pull the sides together at the top before rolling a couple of times to seal. Make sure to leave 3 to 4 inches of "head-room" for the fish.
4. Repeat with the remaining packets, and place all four packets onto a rimmed baking sheet. Bake for 20 minutes.
5. Place each packet on a plate, and cut the packets open at the table to enjoy. Store leftovers in an airtight container in the refrigerator for up to 3 days.

SERVING TIP: Serve these flounder fillets alongside the Brown Rice Pilaf (page 64) or Asparagus and Edamame Salad with citrus vinaigrette (page 53).

PER SERVING: Calories: 224; Total Fat: 4g; Saturated Fat: 1g; Cholesterol: 83mg; Sodium: 118mg; Potassium: 892mg; Carbohydrates: 10g; Fiber: 1g; Sugars: 6g; Protein: 32g

Roasted Herbed Halibut and Vegetables

Serves 6 / Prep time: 10 minutes / Cook time: 20 minutes

Halibut is a firm, mild fish that pairs well with a variety of seasonings and vegetables. Here it's combined with tomatoes and zucchini, but feel free to improvise with what's available in your garden, at the grocery store, or at the farmers' market.

2 small tomatoes, coarsely chopped

2 zucchini, chopped

1 small white onion, chopped

¼ cup coarsely chopped white mushrooms

2 garlic cloves, minced

1 teaspoon herbes de Provence (or a tiny pinch each of dried thyme, marjoram, rosemary, and savory)

½ cup olive oil

Freshly ground black pepper

1 (1½-pound) halibut steak, cut into 6 pieces

3 tablespoons finely chopped fresh tarragon

Juice of 1 lemon

1. Preheat the oven to 350°F.
2. On a large baking sheet, toss the tomatoes, zucchini, onion, mushrooms, garlic, and herbs with the oil, and season with pepper. Arrange the vegetables in a single layer. Roast for 15 to 20 minutes, until soft and slightly browned.
3. Meanwhile, place the halibut steaks on another baking sheet, and season with the tarragon, pepper, and lemon juice. Roast for 10 to 13 minutes, until the fish flakes easily with a fork.
4. Serve the halibut steaks with the roasted vegetables. Store leftovers in an airtight container in the refrigerator for up to 3 days.

SERVING TIP: Add a side of Brown Rice Pilaf (page 64) or Aromatic Almond Couscous (page 65) to bulk up this meal. Make a quick spiced yogurt sauce by combining ½ teaspoon sambal oelek or garlic chili sauce and 1 (6-ounce) container plain nonfat Greek yogurt and serve it over the fish.

PER SERVING: Calories: 288; Total Fat: 20g; Saturated Fat: 3g; Cholesterol: 56mg; Sodium: 85mg; Potassium: 783mg; Carbohydrates: 5g; Fiber: 1g; Sugars: 3g; Protein: 22g

ONE-POT

5 INGREDIENTS OR FEWER

30 MINUTES OR LESS

DAIRY-FREE

GLUTEN-FREE

NUT-FREE

Seared Salmon with Cilantro-Lime Sauce

Serves 4 / Prep time: 5 minutes / Cook time: 15 minutes

Salmon is considered a fatty fish, but don't let the word "fatty" scare you away! It is the best kind of fat for heart health. Just one 6-ounce serving of salmon provides more than half the recommended daily allowance of omega-3 fatty acids. Here it is paired with a bright green sauce that's loaded with flavor.

FOR THE SAUCE

2 garlic cloves, peeled
1½ cups packed fresh cilantro
1 teaspoon grated lime zest

2 tablespoons freshly squeezed lime juice
2 tablespoons olive oil

FOR THE SALMON

Nonstick cooking spray
4 (6-ounce) skin-on salmon fillets

¼ teaspoon freshly ground black pepper

TO MAKE THE SAUCE

1. Put the garlic in a food processor and pulse to mince. Add the cilantro and lime zest and juice and pulse until finely chopped.
2. With the food processor running, drizzle in the oil and process until well combined.

TO MAKE THE SALMON

3. Coat a nonstick skillet with cooking spray and heat it over medium-high heat.
4. Sprinkle the salmon with pepper and place it in the pan skin-side down. Cook until the skin begins to brown, 5 to 6 minutes.

5. Turn the fish over and cook on the other side until the fish is cooked through and flakes easily with a fork, about 6 minutes.
6. Drizzle with the sauce and serve immediately. Store leftovers in an airtight container in the refrigerator for up to 3 days.

SERVING TIP: Serve the salmon with sautéed snap peas for a beautiful spring meal, or with a side of Roasted Balsamic Brussels Sprouts with Pecans (page 63) or Parmesan-Crusted Cauliflower (page 61).

PER SERVING: Calories: 307; Total Fat: 18g; Saturated Fat: 3g; Cholesterol: 94mg; Sodium: 78mg; Potassium: 880mg; Carbohydrates: 1g; Fiber: 0g; Sugars: 0g; Protein: 34g

Pecan-Crusted Honey-Dijon Salmon

Serves 6 / Prep time: 5 minutes / Cook time: 15 minutes

This healthy salmon dish, coated with a pecan–bread crumb mixture, takes less than 20 minutes to prepare, making it a perfect choice for a busy work-day evening. Serve it with quickly sautéed green beans or steamed broccoli and quinoa. You can use walnuts or almonds in place of pecans, if you prefer.

Nonstick cooking spray
3 tablespoons Dijon mustard
1 tablespoon olive oil
1 tablespoon honey
½ cup finely chopped raw unsalted pecans

½ cup plain whole-wheat bread crumbs
6 (4-ounce) salmon fillets
1 tablespoon minced fresh flat-leaf
   parsley, for garnish

1. Preheat the oven to 400°F. Spray a large baking dish lightly with cooking spray.
2. In a small bowl, combine the mustard, oil, and honey. In another small bowl, combine the pecans and bread crumbs.
3. Arrange the fillets in a single layer in the prepared baking dish. Brush each fillet first with the honey-mustard mixture, then top evenly with the pecan mixture.
4. Bake until the salmon is cooked through and flakes easily with a fork, about 15 minutes.
5. Serve immediately, garnished with the parsley. Store leftovers in an airtight container in the refrigerator for up to 3 days.

PER SERVING: Calories: 277; Total Fat: 17g; Saturated Fat: 2g; Cholesterol: 62mg; Sodium: 169mg; Potassium: 619mg; Carbohydrates: 8g; Fiber: 1g; Sugars: 4g; Protein: 24g

Salmon, Black Bean, and Jalapeño Tostadas

Serves 4 / Prep time: 10 minutes / Cook time: 15 minutes

Canned salmon is both convenient and easy on the budget and offers the same health benefits as fresh does. Made with ingredients you're likely to have in your pantry, these quick tostadas are an easy and delicious weeknight dinner.

8 (6-inch) corn tortillas
Nonstick cooking spray
1 (6- to 7-ounce) can no-salt-added boneless, skinless wild Alaskan salmon, drained
1 avocado, diced
2 tablespoons minced pickled jalapeños, plus 2 tablespoons pickling juice, divided

2 cups shredded cabbage
2 tablespoons chopped fresh cilantro
1 (15-ounce) can no-salt-added black beans, drained and rinsed
3 tablespoons reduced-fat sour cream
2 tablespoons prepared pico de gallo
2 scallions, both white and green parts, chopped
Lime wedges, for garnish

1. Preheat the oven to 375°F. Position the racks in the upper and lower thirds of the oven.
2. Spray the tortillas on both sides with cooking spray and arrange them on two baking sheets in a single layer. Bake, rotating and flipping once, until they begin to turn golden, about 12 minutes.
3. Meanwhile, in a medium bowl, mix the salmon, avocado, and jalapeños.
4. In another medium bowl, toss the cabbage, cilantro, and jalapeño pickling juice.
5. In a food processor, combine the beans, sour cream, pico de gallo, and scallions and process until smooth. Transfer the puree to a microwave-safe bowl, cover, and cook on high in the microwave for about 2 minutes, until the mixture is hot.
6. To serve, spread some of the bean mixture on each tortilla. Top with some of the salmon mixture. Place a handful of cabbage slaw on top. Serve garnished with lime wedges. Store leftovers in an airtight container in the refrigerator for 1 to 2 days.

PER SERVING: Calories: 364; Total Fat: 11g; Saturated Fat: 2g; Cholesterol: 24mg; Sodium: 207mg; Potassium: 794mg; Carbohydrates: 50g; Fiber: 13g; Sugars: 3g; Protein: 20g

Clam Spaghetti

Serves 4 / Prep time: 10 minutes / Cook time: 30 minutes

Nothing could be simpler for a weeknight meal than this easy pasta dish, which you can enjoy occasionally on the DASH diet. Clams are rich in iron, protein, omega-3 fatty acids, and vitamin B_{12}.

¼ cup olive oil
1 medium onion, diced
1 medium green bell pepper, diced
4 garlic cloves, minced
½ cup chopped fresh flat-leaf parsley
⅓ teaspoon ground cayenne pepper
Freshly ground black pepper

3 dozen clams
½ cup white wine
8 ounces whole-wheat spaghetti
½ cup freshly grated reduced-fat Parmesan cheese
1 lemon, cut into wedges

1. In a large skillet, heat the oil over medium heat. Add the onion, bell pepper, and garlic and cook until the onion is translucent, 5 to 7 minutes. Add the parsley, cayenne, and black pepper and set aside.
2. Bring a pot of water to a boil. Add the clams and boil for 10 minutes, or until they open. Remove the clams from the pot and shell half of them. Reserve 2 cups of the cooking liquid.
3. Return the skillet to medium-high heat. Add the shelled clam meat to the skillet, along with the remaining clams in their shells, the wine, and 2 cups of the reserved clam cooking liquid. Bring to a simmer, then remove from heat.
4. Meanwhile, in the pot used to cook the clams, cook the pasta until al dente according to the package instructions. Drain and place in a large serving dish.
5. Ladle the clam and vegetable mixture over the pasta and toss. Serve garnished with the Parmesan and lemon wedges. Store leftovers in an airtight container in the refrigerator for 2 to 3 days.

SUBSTITUTION TIP: Use gluten-free noodles, rice- or bean-based pasta, or zucchini noodles to make this dish gluten-free.

PER SERVING: Calories: 431; Total Fat: 15g; Saturated Fat: 3g; Cholesterol: 7mg; Sodium: 334mg; Potassium: 4,478mg; Carbohydrates: 52g; Fiber: 6g; Sugars: 3g; Protein: 21g

Chicken-Asparagus Penne

Serves 4 / Prep time: 10 minutes / Cook time: 25 minutes

Contrasting textures and layers of flavor combine in this pasta dish that's as grati-fying as it is healthful. Mix things up by trying different pasta shapes or switch out the oregano for basil. In place of the asparagus, try fresh green beans or broccoli.

8 ounces whole-wheat penne
8 ounces boneless, skinless chicken breast
1 tablespoon olive oil
½ cup finely chopped white or yellow onion
2 tablespoons minced garlic

4 cups sliced asparagus
4 cups chopped tomatoes
1 teaspoon dried oregano
¼ teaspoon red pepper flakes (optional)
¼ teaspoon freshly ground black pepper

1. Cook the penne until al dente according to the package instructions. Drain and cover to keep warm.
2. While the pasta cooks, pat the chicken dry. Slice the breast crosswise into very thin strips and cut the strips into ½-inch segments.
3. In a large sauté pan or skillet, heat the oil over medium-high heat. Add the chicken and sauté, stirring constantly, until the chicken is lightly browned and cooked through, about 5 minutes. Transfer the chicken to a plate and cover it with foil to keep it warm.
4. Reduce the heat to medium and add the onion and garlic to the pan. Cook, stir-ring occasionally, until the onion is tender, about 3 minutes. Add the asparagus and cook, stirring, until the asparagus is crisp-tender, about 8 minutes.
5. Mix in the tomatoes, oregano, red pepper flakes (if using), and black pepper. Simmer for 5 minutes. Return the chicken to the pan. Cover and simmer until the chicken is warmed through, about 2 minutes.
6. Add the cooked pasta to the pan and toss to coat it with the sauce. Serve warm. Store leftovers in an airtight container in the refrigerator for 3 to 4 days.

PREP TIP: Add ¾ teaspoon salt to this recipe if absolutely necessary for flavor and if it fits within your sodium allowance for the day.

PER SERVING: Calories: 363; Total Fat: 6g; Saturated Fat: 1g; Cholesterol: 32mg; Sodium: 47mg; Potassium: 911mg; Carbohydrates: 58g; Fiber: 10g; Sugars: 8g; Protein: 26g

Spicy Stir-Fried Chicken and Peanuts

Serves 4 / Prep time: 10 minutes / Cook time: 10 minutes

Stir-fry dishes make great weeknight dinners because they're quick to prepare and usually include protein and veggies in one pan. Just add some steamed brown rice or quinoa, and dinner is served.

FOR THE SAUCE

3 tablespoons low-sodium chicken broth
1 tablespoon low-sodium tomato paste
2 teaspoons unseasoned rice vinegar
1 teaspoon granulated sugar

1 teaspoon low-sodium soy sauce
½ teaspoon toasted sesame oil
¼ teaspoon cornstarch
¼ teaspoon red pepper flakes

FOR THE CHICKEN

1 pound boneless, skinless chicken
    breast, cut into 1-inch cubes
1½ teaspoons cornstarch
1 teaspoon rice wine, dry sherry, or
    dry white wine
1 teaspoon low-sodium soy sauce
½ teaspoon minced garlic
1 tablespoon canola oil

2 (½-inch-thick) slices fresh ginger,
    smashed
2 cups sugar snap peas
¼ cup unsalted dry-roasted peanuts,
    for garnish
1 scallion, both white and green parts,
    thinly sliced, for garnish

TO MAKE THE SAUCE

1. In a small bowl, whisk together the broth, tomato paste, vinegar, sugar, soy sauce, sesame oil, cornstarch, and red pepper flakes. Set aside.

TO MAKE THE CHICKEN

2. In a medium bowl, mix together the chicken, cornstarch, wine, soy sauce, and garlic, and stir to coat the chicken thoroughly.
3. In a large sauté pan or skillet, heat the oil over high heat. Add the ginger and cook, stirring, for 10 seconds, until fragrant.

4. Add the chicken, spreading it out into a single layer. Cook, undisturbed, for about 1 minute, just until the chicken begins to brown, then cook, stirring, for 30 seconds more. Spread the chicken out into a single layer again and cook for 30 seconds, then cook, stirring, for 1 to 2 minutes more, until the chicken is lightly browned all over.

5. Stir in the snap peas and cook for 1 minute. Add the sauce and cook, stirring, for about 1 minute, until the sauce thickens and becomes glossy and the chicken is cooked through.

6. Serve immediately, garnished with the peanuts and scallions. Store leftovers in an airtight container in the refrigerator for 3 to 4 days.

PER SERVING: Calories: 244; Total Fat: 11g; Saturated Fat: 1g; Cholesterol: 65mg; Sodium: 144mg; Potassium: 474mg; Carbohydrates: 8g; Fiber: 2g; Sugars: 3g; Protein: 29g

Artichoke-Stuffed Chicken Breasts

Serves 4 / Prep time: 10 minutes / Cook time: 20 minutes

The humble-looking artichoke is one of the most antioxidant-rich foods around and is full of fiber, folate, and vitamins C and K. Goat cheese and lemon are perfect flavor partners; together they turn a plain chicken breast into a feast. For lower sodium content, rinse the artichoke hearts before use.

1 (6-ounce) jar marinated artichoke
    hearts, drained and chopped
1 (3-ounce) package herbed goat cheese,
    at room temperature
2½ tablespoons plain whole-wheat bread
    crumbs

2 teaspoons Italian seasoning
2 teaspoons grated lemon zest
¼ teaspoon freshly ground black pepper
4 (6-ounce) boneless, skinless chicken
    breast halves
Nonstick cooking spray

1. Preheat the oven to 375°F.
2. In a medium bowl, stir together the artichoke hearts, goat cheese, bread crumbs, Italian seasoning, lemon zest, and pepper. Set aside.
3. Place one chicken breast on a piece of plastic wrap on top of a sturdy work surface. Top it with another piece of plastic wrap and, using a meat tenderizing mallet or a rolling pin, pound it to an even thickness of about ¼ inch. Repeat with the remaining chicken breasts.
4. Place about 2 tablespoons of the artichoke-cheese mixture on one end of each of the chicken pieces and roll the chicken up around it. Secure with toothpicks.
5. Coat a large oven-safe sauté pan or skillet with cooking spray and heat over medium-high heat. Add the chicken and cook until browned on both sides, about 3 minutes per side.
6. Transfer the skillet to the preheated oven and bake for about 15 minutes, until the chicken is cooked through. Remove the chicken from the pan and let rest for 5 minutes.
7. Slice each breast in half crosswise and transfer to a serving plate. Serve immediately. Store leftovers in an airtight container in the refrigerator for 3 to 4 days.

PER SERVING: Calories: 283; Total Fat: 9g; Saturated Fat: 4g; Cholesterol: 134mg; Sodium: 200mg; Potassium: 695mg; Carbohydrates: 5g; Fiber: 4g; Sugars: 1g; Protein: 44g

Chicken and Potato Tagine

Serves 6 / Prep time: 10 minutes / Cook time: 60 minutes

The term "tagine" refers to both the cooking vessel and the finished dish. Use a Dutch oven or casserole dish if you don't have a traditional tagine. Small amounts of meat and poultry are balanced with large servings of vegetables on this diet—but watch your intake of potatoes. While this recipe takes a bit of time, it's mostly hands-off.

1 (3-pound) whole chicken, cut into
  8 pieces
1 medium onion, thinly sliced
¼ cup olive oil
3 garlic cloves, minced
1 teaspoon paprika
½ teaspoon ground cumin
½ teaspoon freshly ground black pepper

¼ teaspoon ground ginger
Pinch saffron threads (optional)
2 cups water
3 cups diced peeled potatoes
½ cup chopped fresh flat-leaf parsley
½ cup chopped fresh cilantro
1 cup fresh or frozen green peas

1. In a Dutch oven, combine the chicken, onion, oil, garlic, paprika, cumin, pepper, ginger, and saffron (if using).
2. Add the water and bring to a boil over medium-high heat.
3. Reduce the heat and simmer, covered, for 30 minutes.
4. Add the potatoes, parsley, and cilantro, and simmer an additional 20 minutes, or until the potatoes are almost tender. Add the peas at the last moment and simmer for an additional 5 minutes.
5. Serve hot. Store leftovers in an airtight container in the refrigerator for 3 to 4 days.

INGREDIENT TIP: Saffron can be a pricey spice, but it's worth every ounce of flavor it provides.

PER SERVING: Calories: 465; Total Fat: 30g; Saturated Fat: 7g; Cholesterol: 104mg; Sodium: 130mg; Potassium: 691mg; Carbohydrates: 19g; Fiber: 3g; Sugars: 3g; Protein: 29g

Grilled Chicken and Vegetables in Lemon-Walnut Sauce

Serves 4 / Prep time: 10 minutes / Cook time: 20 minutes

This grilled chicken and vegetable dish gets a boost from a rich pureed walnut sauce. Other vegetables, such as artichokes, carrots, eggplant, or endive, can be used in place of, or in addition to, the zucchini and asparagus. If you don't have a grill, you can make it on the stovetop in a grill pan.

1 cup chopped raw unsalted walnuts, toasted
1 small shallot, finely chopped
½ cup olive oil, plus more for brushing
Grated zest and juice of 1 lemon
4 boneless, skinless chicken breasts

Freshly ground black pepper
2 zucchini, sliced diagonally ¼ inch thick
8 ounces asparagus, trimmed
1 red onion, sliced ⅓ inch thick
1 teaspoon Italian seasoning

1. Heat a grill to medium-high.
2. In a food processor, combine the walnuts, shallot, oil, lemon zest, and lemon juice and process until smooth and creamy.
3. Lightly oil the grill grates. Season the chicken with pepper and grill for 7 to 8 minutes on the first side, then turn.
4. Put the zucchini, asparagus, and onion on the grill with the chicken. Sprinkle the Italian seasoning to taste over the chicken and vegetables and cook for 7 to 8 minutes more, until the vegetables are tender and an instant-read thermometer inserted into the thickest part of the chicken reaches 165°F.
5. To serve, lay the grilled veggies on a plate, place the chicken breast on the vegetables, and spoon the walnut sauce over the chicken and vegetables. Store leftovers in an airtight container in the refrigerator for 3 to 4 days.

SUBSTITUTION TIP: If you're having trouble finding unsalted toasted walnuts, simply toast your own (see page 34).

PER SERVING: Calories: 644; Total Fat: 50g; Saturated Fat: 6g; Cholesterol: 103mg; Sodium: 75mg; Potassium: 934mg; Carbohydrates: 13g; Fiber: 5g; Sugars: 6g; Protein: 39g

Pomegranate-Glazed Chicken

Serves 6 / Prep time: 10 minutes / Cook time: 30 minutes

In this recipe, the pomegranate juice makes a sweet, fruity glaze for boneless, skinless chicken breasts. From start to finish, this dish takes less than 30 minutes to prepare. Look for no-sugar-added pomegranate juice. Serve with Tuscan Kale Salad Massaged with Roasted Garlic (page 54) for a decadent dinner.

6 tablespoons olive oil, divided
1 teaspoon ground cumin
1 garlic clove, minced
Freshly ground black pepper
6 boneless, skinless chicken breasts
1 cup no-sugar-added pomegranate juice

2 tablespoons honey
1 tablespoon Dijon mustard
½ teaspoon dried thyme
Seeds from 1 pomegranate, or 1 cup
   pomegranate seeds

1. In a small bowl, mix 2 tablespoons of the oil, the cumin, garlic, and pepper and rub it into the chicken.
2. In a large skillet, heat the remaining 4 tablespoons oil over medium heat. Add the chicken breasts and sauté for 10 minutes, turning once halfway through, until the chicken breasts are golden brown on each side.
3. Add the pomegranate juice, honey, mustard, and thyme.
4. Reduce the heat and simmer for 20 minutes, or until the chicken is cooked through and the sauce reduces by half.
5. Transfer the chicken and sauce to a serving platter, top with the pomegranate seeds, and serve. Store leftovers in an airtight container in the refrigerator for 3 to 4 days.

PER SERVING: Calories: 410; Total Fat: 19g; Saturated Fat: 3g; Cholesterol: 124mg; Sodium: 112mg; Potassium: 784mg; Carbohydrates: 20g; Fiber: 2g; Sugars: 17g; Protein: 39g

Wild Rice and Chicken-Stuffed Tomatoes

Serves 4 / Prep time: 15 minutes / Cook time: 20 minutes

If you want to add a little extra flavor to this dish, you can cook the wild rice in low-sodium chicken or vegetable broth. Make sure you read the label on the broth carefully, because some reduced-sodium products still contain a large amount of salt. Use 2 cups of broth to 1 cup of rice for the best results.

4 large tomatoes
2 cups cooked wild rice
8 ounces cooked boneless, skinless chicken breast, chopped
½ cup grated reduced-fat Parmesan cheese

¼ cup chopped unsalted pistachios
1 celery stalk, finely chopped
4 teaspoons chopped fresh basil
2 teaspoons minced garlic
2 teaspoons olive oil
Freshly ground black pepper

1. Preheat the oven to 350°F.
2. Carefully cut the tops off the tomatoes and scoop out the insides with a spoon, leaving an intact shell and reserving the interior pulp. Place the tomato shells in a shallow baking dish.
3. Chop the reserved tomato pulp coarsely and transfer to a medium bowl.
4. Add the cooked rice, chicken, cheese, pistachios, celery, basil, and garlic to the tomato pulp and mix well.
5. Spoon the filling evenly into the tomato shells. Drizzle the stuffed tomatoes with the oil.
6. Bake the stuffed tomatoes until the filling is piping hot and the tomatoes are softened but not collapsed, about 20 minutes.
7. Season with pepper and serve. Store leftovers in an airtight container in the refrigerator for 3 to 4 days.

SUBSTITUTION TIP: For a vegetarian version of the recipe, replace the chicken with a 15-ounce can of no-salt-added chickpeas or lentils, drained and rinsed.

PER SERVING: Calories: 277; Total Fat: 10g; Saturated Fat: 3g; Cholesterol: 43mg; Sodium: 236mg; Potassium: 769mg; Carbohydrates: 28g; Fiber: 5g; Sugars: 6g; Protein: 22g

Turkey Lettuce Cups

Serves 4 / Prep time: 15 minutes / Cook time: 10 minutes

Bibb lettuce is a tender but crisp, fresh alternative to bread or tortillas that adds a brightness to this recipe. You may find that using lettuce to make cups or wraps is a new favorite method in your home, with the added benefit of increasing your vegetable intake.

2 teaspoons toasted sesame oil
20 ounces lean ground turkey
1 tablespoon minced fresh ginger
1 (12-ounce) can no-salt-added baby corn, drained and chopped into 1-inch pieces
1 (8-ounce) can no-salt-added water chestnuts, drained and chopped

1 cup snap peas cut in 1-inch pieces
½ cup low-sodium chicken broth
4 scallions, both white and green parts, minced
2 tablespoons hoisin sauce
8 Bibb lettuce leaves
½ cup chopped fresh cilantro
1 carrot, shredded

1. In a large nonstick pan, heat the oil over medium-high heat. Add the turkey and ginger and cook, crumbling the meat with a wooden spoon, until the turkey is cooked through, about 8 minutes.
2. Stir in the baby corn, water chestnuts, snap peas, broth, scallions, and hoisin sauce. Cook for 1 minute more.
3. Spoon some of the turkey mixture into each lettuce leaf, top with the cilantro and carrot, and roll into wraps. Serve immediately. Store leftover turkey mixture and lettuce leaves in separate airtight containers in the refrigerator for 3 to 4 days.

PREP TIP: Purchase shredded carrots to make this even easier, or buy a frozen blend of stir-fry veggies and thaw it before using.

PER SERVING: Calories: 420; Total Fat: 15g; Saturated Fat: 4g; Cholesterol: 105mg; Sodium: 247mg; Potassium: 838mg; Carbohydrates: 42g; Fiber: 4g; Sugars: 4g; Protein: 32g

ONE-POT

30 MINUTES OR LESS

DAIRY-FREE

NUT-FREE

Herbed Turkey Medallions with Rice

Serves 4 / Prep time: 5 minutes / Cook time: 1 hour 10 minutes

Turkey is not just for Thanksgiving! Turkey breast is actually leaner than chicken breast and can be a delicious alternative to chicken on the menu. This recipe is simple to make in larger batches, providing great leftovers or freezer meals. Cut down on prep and overall time by using microwavable frozen rice packets, which can be found in the freezer aisles of most grocery stores.

1 teaspoon olive oil

4 (6-ounce) turkey breast cutlets

1 cup thinly sliced yellow onion

1 cup low-sodium chicken broth

1 tablespoon chopped fresh sage or dried sage

1 tablespoon chopped fresh rosemary or dried rosemary

½ teaspoon freshly ground black pepper

1 tablespoon cornstarch

½ cup dry white wine

4 cups water

2 cups short-grain brown rice

1. In a large heavy skillet, heat the oil over medium-high heat. Add the turkey and brown for about 5 minutes on each side, then add the onion, broth, sage, rosemary, and pepper.
2. In a small bowl, stir the cornstarch into the wine until smooth, then whisk the mixture into the skillet with the turkey. Reduce the heat to low and simmer for 15 to 20 minutes, until the turkey is cooked through.
3. Meanwhile, in medium pot, combine the water and rice. Bring to a simmer over medium-high heat, then reduce the heat to low, cover, and cook for 45 to 50 minutes, until the water is absorbed.
4. Fluff the rice with a fork and serve with the turkey. Store leftovers in an airtight container in the refrigerator for 3 to 4 days.

PER SERVING: Calories: 593; Total Fat: 8g; Saturated Fat: 1g; Cholesterol: 90mg; Sodium: 133mg; Potassium: 776mg; Carbohydrates: 78g; Fiber: 4g; Sugars: 2g; Protein: 47g

Simple Turkey Meatloaf

Serves 4 / Prep time: 10 minutes / Cook time: 45 minutes

Moist, savory turkey meatloaf is wonderful comfort food. All the more comforting is the money you save when you buy ground turkey instead of ground beef. Make sure to read the labels and use the leanest grade you can find—at least 90 percent lean. The leaner the ground turkey, the higher the proportion of white meat to dark meat and the less skin it will contain.

1 teaspoon canola oil

1 pound lean ground turkey

½ cup old-fashioned oats

½ cup chopped white or yellow onion

1 large egg

4 teaspoons chopped fresh flat-leaf parsley

1 tablespoon Worcestershire sauce

¾ teaspoon freshly ground black pepper

5 tablespoons low-sodium ketchup, divided

1. Preheat the oven to 350°F. Use the oil to grease the bottom of a 9-by-13-inch baking pan.
2. In a large bowl, combine the turkey, oats, onion, egg, parsley, Worcestershire, pepper, and 3 tablespoons of the ketchup. Using your hands, thoroughly mix the ingredients.
3. Form the turkey mixture into a 9-by-5-inch oval loaf. Place the loaf in the middle of the prepared baking pan. Brush the loaf with the remaining 2 tablespoons ketchup.
4. Bake the meatloaf for about 45 minutes, until internal temperature of the meatloaf reaches 165°F and no pink remains.
5. Slice the meatloaf into quarters and serve. Store leftovers in an airtight container in the refrigerator for 3 to 4 days.

PER SERVING: Calories: 270; Total Fat: 12g; Saturated Fat: 3g; Cholesterol: 130mg; Sodium: 144mg; Potassium: 425mg; Carbohydrates: 15g; Fiber: 2g; Sugars: 6g; Protein: 24g

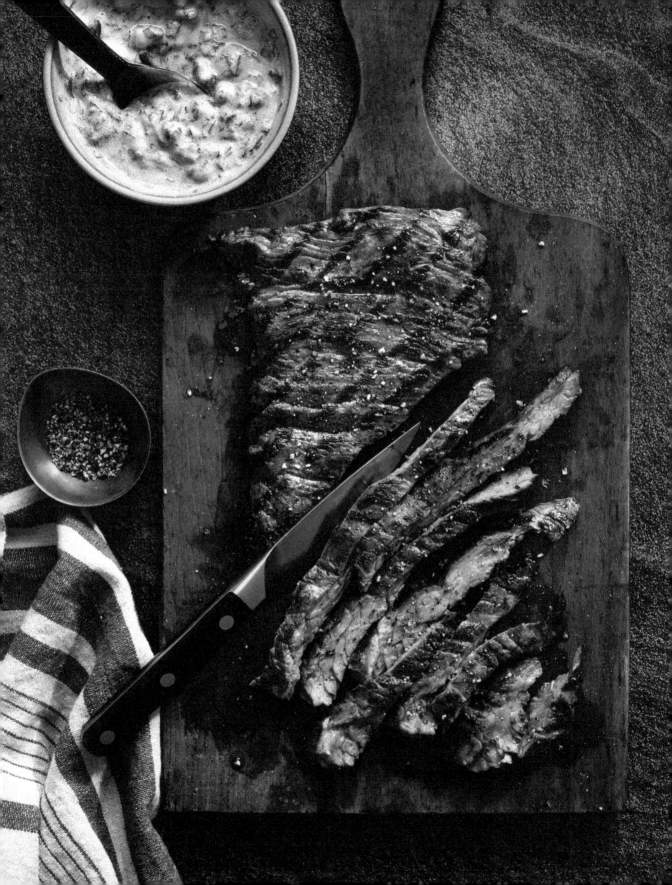

CHAPTER SIX

Beef and Pork Mains

Afelia (Red Wine-Marinated Pork)

Serves 6 / Prep time: 10 minutes, plus several hours or overnight to marinate / Cook time: 2 hours 25 minutes

Afelia gets its unique flavor from coriander, cinnamon, and red wine. Red wine is antioxidant rich, but if you choose not to consume alcohol, you can substitute it with equal parts beef or chicken broth, or red wine vinegar. Afelia is delicious atop brown rice and served with a green salad. Leftovers are also versatile as a pita or wrap.

2 pounds boneless pork roast, cut into 2-inch pieces
1 cup red wine
1 tablespoon crushed coriander seeds
1 cinnamon stick

Freshly ground black pepper
¼ cup olive oil
1 cup small white onions, peeled
3 bay leaves

1. Put the pork chunks in a shallow bowl or zip-top bag. Add the wine, coriander seeds, and cinnamon stick and marinate for several hours or overnight.
2. Drain, reserving the marinade, and pat the pork chunks dry with a paper towel. Season the pork with pepper.
3. In a large stew pot or skillet, heat the oil over medium-high heat. Add the pork and onions and cook, stirring frequently, for 8 to 10 minutes, until browned.
4. Add the bay leaves, more pepper, and the reserved marinade. Cover and simmer on low for 2 hours, or until the pork is very tender.
5. Remove the lid and simmer for an additional 15 minutes to thicken the sauce, then serve. Store leftovers in an airtight container in the refrigerator for 3 to 4 days.

SERVING TIP: Serve with Parmesan-Crusted Cauliflower (page 61), Brown Rice Pilaf (page 64), or Aromatic Almond Couscous (page 65) for a more substantial meal.

PER SERVING: Calories: 282; Total Fat: 15g; Saturated Fat: 3g; Cholesterol: 97mg; Sodium: 72mg; Potassium: 558mg; Carbohydrates: 1g; Fiber: 1g; Sugars: 1g; Protein: 32g

Roasted Spiced Pork Tenderloin

**Serves 6 / Prep time: 10 minutes, plus several hours or overnight to marinate /
Cook time: 15 minutes, plus 15 minutes to rest**

By simply altering the seasonings slightly, this traditional pork tenderloin takes on a decidedly Spanish flair. Remember, the diet recommends 6 ounces of lean poultry or fish per day, including lean pork. Serve it with red potatoes, or add it to salads, wraps, or sandwiches.

2 tablespoons olive oil
1 teaspoon Spanish paprika
1 teaspoon red wine vinegar
1 garlic clove, minced
½ teaspoon ground cumin
½ teaspoon ground coriander

½ teaspoon ground ginger
½ teaspoon freshly ground black pepper
¼ teaspoon ground turmeric
1 pound pork tenderloin
Freshly ground black pepper

1. In a small bowl, combine the oil, paprika, vinegar, garlic, cumin, coriander, ginger, pepper, and turmeric to make a thick paste.
2. Spread the marinade over the pork, set on a plate, cover, and refrigerate for several hours or up to overnight.
3. Heat a grill to medium. Grill the tenderloin for 10 to 12 minutes, turning once halfway through, until an instant-read thermometer inserted into the tenderloin reads 145°F.
4. Transfer the meat to a plate and allow it to rest for 15 minutes before slicing. Slice, season with pepper to taste, and serve. Store leftovers in an airtight container in the refrigerator for 3 to 4 days.

PREP TIP: If you don't have a grill, sear the pork on all sides on the stovetop, then roast in the oven at 375°F for 20 to 25 minutes.

PER SERVING: Calories: 134; Total Fat: 7g; Saturated Fat: 2g; Cholesterol: 49mg; Sodium: 40mg; Potassium: 315mg; Carbohydrates: 1g; Fiber: 1g; Sugars: 1g; Protein: 16g

ONE-POT

DAIRY-FREE

GLUTEN-FREE

NUT-FREE

Honey-Mustard Pork Chops

Serves 2 / Prep time: 10 minutes / Cook time: 35 minutes

This is one of my personal favorite pork preparations (it also works perfectly with chicken or salmon). Pork chops, when trimmed of the fat, are an excellent lean protein source on the DASH diet. The Dijon mustard and honey caramelize perfectly, and the panko adds a pleasing crunch.

Nonstick cooking spray
½ cup whole-wheat panko bread crumbs
1 tablespoon cornstarch
1 teaspoon paprika

1 teaspoon chili powder
2 tablespoons Dijon mustard
1 tablespoon honey
2 boneless lean pork chops

1. Preheat the oven to 375°F. Lightly coat a baking dish with cooking spray.
2. In a shallow bowl, mix the bread crumbs, cornstarch, paprika, and chili powder together.
3. In another bowl, mix the mustard and honey together.
4. Dip the pork chops into the honey-mustard mixture and then into the bread crumb mixture to coat.
5. Set the pork chops in the baking dish and bake, uncovered, for 35 minutes, or until an instant-read thermometer registers at 145°F and the juices run clear. Store leftovers in an airtight container in the refrigerator for 3 to 4 days.

SERVING TIP: Serve with a side of Maple-Pecan Mashed Sweet Potatoes (page 62) or Roasted Balsamic Brussels Sprouts with Pecans (page 63), if desired.

PER SERVING: Calories: 338; Total Fat: 11g; Saturated Fat: 4g; Cholesterol: 95mg; Sodium: 378mg; Potassium: 637mg; Carbohydrates: 24g; Fiber: 2g; Sugars: 10g; Protein: 33g

Pork Loin with Dried Fig Sauce

Serves 6 / Prep time: 20 minutes / Cook time: 55 minutes, plus 15 minutes to rest

Imagining this recipe on my table makes my mouth water. The natural sweetness of the carrots and figs pairs beautifully with the savory herbs and tender pork loin. This recipe is sure to draw a crowd, so you can always double it.

1 tablespoon chopped fresh rosemary
1 tablespoon chopped fresh thyme
Freshly ground black pepper
1 (3-pound) pork loin
½ cup olive oil
3 carrots, sliced

1 onion, diced
1 garlic clove, minced
1 cup dried figs, cut into small pieces
1 cup white wine or white wine vinegar
Juice of 1 lemon

1. Preheat the oven to 300°F.
2. In a small bowl, mix the rosemary, thyme, and pepper together to make a dry rub. Press the rub into the pork loin.
3. In a large skillet, heat the oil over medium-high heat. Add the pork loin, carrots, onion, and garlic and cook for 15 minutes, or until the pork is browned on all sides.
4. Transfer the pork and vegetables to a shallow roasting pan. Add the figs, wine, and lemon juice.
5. Cover with foil and bake for 40 to 50 minutes, until the meat is tender and the internal temperature is 145°F.
6. Transfer the meat to a serving dish and cover with foil. Let rest for 15 minutes before slicing.
7. In the meantime, pour the vegetables, figs, and liquids into a blender. Blend until smooth and strain through a sieve or strainer.
8. Transfer to a gravy dish to pass at the table or pour directly over the sliced meat before serving. Store leftovers in an airtight container in the refrigerator for 3 to 4 days.

INGREDIENT TIP: If you can't find dried figs, substitute dried apricots instead. Both dried figs and dried apricots are high in fiber. Serve with a green salad for a delicious, well-rounded dinner.

PER SERVING: Calories: 576; Total Fat: 28g; Saturated Fat: 5g; Cholesterol: 143mg; Sodium: 138mg; Potassium: 1,184mg; Carbohydrates: 22g; Fiber: 4g; Sugars: 15g; Protein: 52g

Boneless Pork Chops with Curried Apples

Serves 4 / Prep time: 5 minutes / Cook time: 25 minutes

Pork and apples are a classic flavor pairing that is a winner for a reason. This recipe is sure to make its way onto your regular menu, not to mention how quickly it comes together with staple pantry ingredients.

2 tablespoons olive oil
4 lean boneless pork chops
1 large yellow onion, coarsely chopped
4 medium apples, peeled, cored, and thinly sliced

1 cup unsweetened apple juice
2 to 3 tablespoons curry powder
Freshly ground black pepper
8 ounces whole-wheat pasta

1. In a large heavy sauté pan or skillet, heat the oil over medium-high heat. Add the pork chops and brown on the first side for 1 to 2 minutes, then flip the chops and brown on the other side for 1 to 2 minutes. Transfer the pork to a plate and set aside.
2. Add the onion to the skillet. Reduce the heat to low and cook until just softened, 8 to 10 minutes. Add the apples, apple juice, and curry powder and mix thoroughly. Season with pepper. Increase the heat to maintain a gentle simmer and cook for 10 minutes. Return the pork to the skillet, cover with the apples, and cook for 10 minutes, or until the meat is tender and an instant-read thermometer registers 145°F. (If the sauce is too thin, remove the pork and cook on high for 1 to 2 minutes to reduce it; if the sauce is too thick, add 1 to 2 tablespoons water.)
3. Meanwhile, cook the pasta according to the package instructions. Drain.
4. Divide the noodles among four plates. Place a pork chop on top of each and cover with the curried apples. Serve immediately. Store leftovers in an airtight container in the refrigerator for 3 to 4 days.

PER SERVING: Calories: 640; Total Fat: 15g; Saturated Fat: 3g; Cholesterol: 122mg; Sodium: 103mg; Potassium: 1,187mg; Carbohydrates: 80g; Fiber: 11g; Sugars: 27g; Protein: 51g

Pork Chops
and Garlic Sweet Potatoes

Serves 2 / Prep time: 10 minutes / Cook time: 40 minutes

Sweet potatoes are rich in vitamins and minerals, particularly vitamin A, which is a potent antioxidant. You may be most familiar with sweet potatoes, cousin to the yam, at Thanksgiving with marshmallows on top, but featured in this recipe, roasted with garlic, they make the perfect base layer for the pork chops.

2 large sweet potatoes
1 tablespoon minced garlic
Dried or chopped fresh sage
Freshly ground black pepper

2 lean boneless pork chops
Dry mustard powder
1 cup skim milk

1. Preheat the oven to 375°F.
2. Slice the potatoes into ½-inch-thick slices and toss them in a bowl with the garlic. Season lightly with sage and pepper.
3. Spread the potatoes in a nonstick baking pan and top with the pork chops.
4. Dust the pork chops lightly with dry mustard and then pour the milk into the pan and onto the potatoes.
5. Cover and bake for 30 minutes, then uncover and bake for another 10 minutes, until the meat is tender and the internal temperature is 145°F. Store leftovers in an airtight container in the refrigerator for 3 to 4 days.

PREP TIP: If you have fresh herbs on hand, add a few snips of rosemary, thyme, or tarragon.

PER SERVING: Calories: 342; Total Fat: 5g; Saturated Fat: 2g; Cholesterol: 86mg; Sodium: 206mg; Potassium: 1,212mg; Carbohydrates: 34g; Fiber: 4g; Sugars: 11g; Protein: 38g

Hoisin Pork and Veggie Stir-Fry

Serves 4 / Prep time: 15 minutes / Cook time: 15 minutes

Stir-fry is a simple, quick, vegetable-packed dish that incorporates sweet, savory, tangy, and pleasantly bitter flavors. The hoisin sauce delectably coats the pork and vegetables, also making a delicious sauce.

¼ cup hoisin sauce

1 tablespoon mirin, dry sherry, or dry white wine

1 tablespoon plus 2 teaspoons toasted sesame oil, divided

1 tablespoon grated peeled fresh ginger

2 garlic cloves, minced

1½ pounds pork tenderloin, thinly sliced

1 shallot, thinly sliced

2 cups shredded napa cabbage

1 red bell pepper, cut into matchsticks

1 cup snow peas, sliced on the diagonal

1 tablespoon cornstarch, mixed with 1 tablespoon cold water

4 scallions, both white and green parts, thinly sliced on the diagonal, for garnish

2 tablespoons toasted sesame seeds, for garnish

1. In a large zip-top bag, combine the hoisin sauce, mirin, 1 tablespoon of the oil, ginger, and garlic. Seal and shake to incorporate. Add the pork, seal, and toss to coat well, then let sit for 15 minutes.
2. In a large sauté pan or skillet, heat the remaining 2 teaspoons oil over medium-high heat. Add the shallot and cook, stirring, until it begins to soften, about 3 minutes.
3. Remove the pork from the marinade, reserving the marinade. Add the pork and cook, stirring, for 1 minute. Add the cabbage, bell pepper, and snow peas and cook, stirring, until the vegetables begin to soften, about 3 minutes.
4. Stir in the reserved marinade and bring to a boil. Cook, stirring, until the sauce begins to thicken, about 3 minutes. Add the cornstarch mixture and cook, stirring, until the sauce has thickened, about 2 minutes.
5. Serve immediately, garnished with the scallions and sesame seeds. Store leftovers in an airtight container in the refrigerator for 3 to 4 days.

PER SERVING: Calories: 351; Total Fat: 14g; Saturated Fat: 3g; Cholesterol: 111mg; Sodium: 379mg; Potassium: 951mg; Carbohydrates: 16g; Fiber: 3g; Sugars: 7g; Protein: 38g

Buffalo Burgers

Serves 4 / Prep time: 15 minutes / Cook time: 10 minutes

While consumed infrequently in America, buffalo meat is extremely lean and has a beef-like flavor and texture. Due to its lean nature, it can be cooked for less time than beef, so it stays as moist as possible. You may just find that ground buffalo is a new house favorite for burgers, tacos, and in any recipe that calls for ground beef. To lower the sodium content of this recipe, omit the cheese or serve these burgers "protein style" (without a bun).

1 pound ground buffalo (American bison) meat

½ yellow onion, minced

¼ cup smoky barbecue sauce, such as chipotle-honey, plus more for serving

1 teaspoon freshly ground black pepper

1 teaspoon smoked paprika

8 spelt bread slices or 4 spelt buns

4 slices smoked low-fat mozzarella cheese

1. Heat a grill to medium.
2. In a large bowl, combine the buffalo, onion, barbecue sauce, pepper, and paprika, until well mixed. Shape into four patties.
3. Place the patties on the grill and sear for about 3 minutes per side, or until cooked through.
4. Serve on spelt bread, topped with cheese and additional barbecue sauce. Store leftovers in an airtight container in the refrigerator for 3 to 4 days.

SERVING TIP: Dress up your burger with lettuce, onion, pickle, tomato, or your favorite burger toppings.

PER SERVING: Calories: 352; Total Fat: 8g; Saturated Fat: 4g; Cholesterol: 70mg; Sodium: 578mg; Potassium: 534mg; Carbohydrates: 34g; Fiber: 3g; Sugars: 7g; Protein: 35g

ONE-POT

30 MINUTES OR LESS

NUT-FREE

Beef Tostadas

Serves 4 / Prep time: 10 minutes / Cook time: 15 minutes

Tostadas, tacos, nachos, and burritos are a huge hit in my house, and they are amazingly simple to make DASH-diet friendly. All you need is a whole-grain base (corn shell or whole-wheat tortilla), a lean protein, herbs and spices, no-salt-added beans, veggies, and low-fat cheese, and you can make a Tex-Mex dinner with ease in under 30 minutes.

1 tablespoon olive oil
8 ounces lean ground beef
½ teaspoon ground cumin
½ teaspoon freshly ground black pepper
½ teaspoon chili powder
1 (15-ounce) can no-salt-added black beans, drained and rinsed
6 tablespoons no-salt-added tomato paste

4 crispy tostada shells
2 cups shredded reduced-fat Mexican-style cheese blend
2 cups shredded lettuce
2 cups chopped fresh tomato
¾ cup diced white onion
¼ cup black olives, sliced

1. Lightly coat a heavy sauté pan or skillet with the oil and heat over medium-high heat. Add the beef and cook until browned.
2. Season with the cumin, pepper, and chili powder. Cook for 10 minutes, until the beef is cooked through, then add the black beans and tomato paste and stir well. Reduce the heat to low and cover to keep warm.
3. Place one tostada shell on each plate and top with one-quarter of the beef mixture. Top with the shredded cheese, then the lettuce, tomato, onion, and olives. Store leftovers in airtight containers, with the meat and fresh ingredients stored separately, in the refrigerator for 3 to 4 days.

SERVING TIP: Add sliced avocado or jalapeños, salsa (store-bought or homemade; see page 76), or your other favorite toppings to this recipe.

PER SERVING: Calories: 494; Total Fat: 24g; Saturated Fat: 10g; Cholesterol: 72mg; Sodium: 647mg; Potassium: 1,071mg; Carbohydrates: 37g; Fiber: 10g; Sugars: 7g; Protein: 34g

Spicy Lettuce-Wrapped Beef

Serves 4 / Prep time: 15 minutes / Cook time: 15 minutes

Lettuce wraps are a crisp, fresh alternative to tortilla wraps that increase your vegetable intake on the DASH diet. The meaty steak and medley of herbs and spices are complemented by the lettuce, rather than hidden underneath a heavy tortilla.

1 pound flank steak
¼ teaspoon freshly ground black pepper
½ seedless cucumber, peeled and diced
6 cherry tomatoes, halved
1 shallot, thinly sliced
1 tablespoon finely chopped fresh mint

1 tablespoon finely chopped fresh basil
1 tablespoon finely chopped fresh cilantro
2 tablespoons low-sodium soy sauce
2 tablespoons freshly squeezed lime juice
½ teaspoon red pepper flakes
1 head Bibb lettuce, leaves separated

1. Heat a grill to medium-high or heat a grill pan over medium-high heat.
2. Sprinkle the steak with pepper on both sides. Grill the steak, turning once, until the desired degree of doneness has been reached, about 7 minutes per side for medium-rare.
3. Transfer the steak to a cutting board, cover loosely with foil, and let rest for 5 minutes. Cut into ¼-inch-thick slices across the grain.
4. In a large bowl, mix together the sliced steak, cucumber, tomatoes, shallot, mint, basil, and cilantro.
5. In a small bowl, whisk together the soy sauce, lime juice, and red pepper flakes. Pour the dressing over the steak mixture and toss to coat.
6. To serve, place the meat mixture in a serving bowl with a large spoon. Set the lettuce leaves on a serving plate and instruct diners to scoop some of the meat into a lettuce leaf, wrap it up like a burrito, and enjoy. Store leftovers in airtight containers, with the meat and lettuce wraps stored separately, in the refrigerator for 3 to 4 days.

SERVING TIP: Serve with bowls of extra condiments, like chopped fresh herbs, sliced chiles, chili paste, Asian-style pickles, or kimchi, if you like.

PER SERVING: Calories: 211; Total Fat: 10g; Saturated Fat: 4g; Cholesterol: 77mg; Sodium: 322mg; Potassium: 639mg; Carbohydrates: 5g; Fiber: 1g; Sugars: 2g; Protein: 26g

30 MINUTES OR LESS

DAIRY-FREE

NUT-FREE

Orange Beef and Stir-Fried Vegetables

Serves 4 / Prep time: 10 minutes / Cook time: 10 minutes

This tangy-sweet recipe calls for hoisin sauce, which is readily available in the Asian section of your supermarket. Fragrant, sweet, and salty, hoisin is a common component in Asian marinades and stir-fries and is also used as a dipping sauce. Stir-frying is a lightning-fast cooking technique, so make sure you have all your ingredients prepped and nearby before you turn on the stove.

½ cup freshly squeezed orange juice
1 tablespoon cornstarch
3 tablespoons hoisin sauce
1 tablespoon low-sodium soy sauce
1 tablespoon dry sherry (optional)
1 tablespoon canola oil
1 tablespoon minced garlic

1 tablespoon minced peeled fresh ginger
12 ounces flank steak, sliced across the
   grain into thin strips
1 cup broccoli florets
1 red bell pepper, cut into thin strips
2 celery stalks, sliced crosswise
½ cup sliced shiitake mushrooms

1. In a medium bowl, stir together the orange juice and cornstarch until smooth. Whisk in the hoisin, soy sauce, and sherry (if using). Set aside.
2. Heat a large skillet over medium-high heat. Add the oil and heat until it is hot but not smoking. Add the garlic and ginger and cook, stirring quickly and constantly, for 30 seconds to 1 minute.
3. Add the beef and stir-fry until the meat loses its redness, about 2 minutes. Transfer the beef, garlic, and ginger to a bowl and set aside.
4. Add the broccoli to the skillet and stir-fry until it is bright green, about 2 minutes. Add the bell pepper and celery and stir-fry for 1 minute. Add the mushrooms and stir-fry for 2 minutes.
5. Form a well in the center of the vegetables and pour in the orange-hoisin mixture. When the liquid reaches a boil, reduce the heat to medium-low.

6. Return the beef to the pan and mix thoroughly with the vegetables and sauce. Cook for about 1 minute, until the sauce thickens.
7. Serve immediately. Store leftovers in an airtight container in the refrigerator for 3 to 4 days.

INGREDIENT TIP: Use whatever additional vegetables you'd like or that you have on hand in this stir-fry, including cauliflower, snow peas, and carrots.

PER SERVING: Calories: 249; Total Fat: 11g; Saturated Fat: 3g; Cholesterol: 58mg; Sodium: 394mg; Potassium: 592mg; Carbohydrates: 16g; Fiber: 2g; Sugars: 8g; Protein: 20g

Pot Roast with Sweet Potatoes, Peas, and Onions

Serves 6 / Prep time: 10 minutes / Cook time: 4 hours

While this recipe may appear daunting, it's mostly hands-off cooking as the pot roast cooks in a large amount of liquid, almost creating a stew. Serve the melt-in-your-mouth beef in a bowl with the juices and vegetables.

1 (3- to 4-pound) beef pot roast
Freshly ground black pepper
1 tablespoon olive oil
1 (14.5-ounce) can low-sodium beef broth
1 cup red wine
1 large onion, diced
1 carrot, cut into 1-inch-thick coins
2 garlic cloves, chopped
1 cinnamon stick

3 large sweet potatoes, peeled and diced into 1-inch cubes
1 (10-ounce) package frozen peas
½ cup chopped fresh flat-leaf parsley leaves
¼ cup chopped fresh rosemary and/or thyme leaves
Juice of ½ lemon

1. Rinse the roast under cold running water and pat dry with paper towels. Roll the roast in pepper on all sides.
2. In a large stockpot, heat the oil over medium-high heat. Add the roast and cook, turning every few minutes, until browned on all sides, about 8 minutes. Remove the pot from the heat.
3. Pour the broth and wine over the beef. Add the onion, carrot, garlic, and cinnamon stick to the pot and enough water to cover the meat. Bring to a boil over high heat, then reduce the heat to medium and simmer for 3 hours, adding more water or broth as needed, until the beef is falling apart.
4. Add the sweet potatoes and simmer for 30 minutes. Add the peas and cook for 10 minutes.
5. Remove the pan from the heat. Stir in the parsley, rosemary, and lemon juice. Transfer the roast to a deep platter and spoon the vegetables and liquid around it. Serve immediately. Store leftovers in an airtight container in the refrigerator for 3 to 4 days.

PER SERVING: Calories: 621; Total Fat: 34g; Saturated Fat: 14g; Cholesterol: 150mg; Sodium: 270mg; Potassium: 1,152mg; Carbohydrates: 25g; Fiber: 5g; Sugars: 7g; Protein: 48g

Spaghetti with Meat Sauce

Serves 6 / Prep time: 5 minutes / Cook time: 40 minutes

Ground beef comes in a variety of lean options, up to 93 percent lean, making it as lean, or leaner, than ground turkey. This recipe is the perfect example of how the DASH diet can incorporate your favorite meals and comfort foods, and you will find that you do not even miss the added salt and fat.

2 tablespoons olive oil
1 cup finely chopped white or yellow onion
3 garlic cloves, minced
1 pound lean ground beef
½ teaspoon salt (optional)
1 (28-ounce) can no-salt-added crushed
  tomatoes

1 tablespoon balsamic vinegar
2 teaspoons dried oregano
2 teaspoons dried basil
1 teaspoon freshly ground
  black pepper
12 ounces whole-wheat
  spaghetti

1. In a large sauté pan or skillet, heat the oil over medium-high heat. Add the onion and garlic and cook, stirring, until the onion softens, about 5 minutes.
2. Add the beef and salt (if using), and brown, breaking up the chunks, for 5 minutes. Using a slotted spoon, transfer the beef mixture to a bowl, leaving behind the fat.
3. In a large saucepan, combine the drained beef mixture, tomatoes, vinegar, oregano, basil, and pepper over medium-high heat. Bring the sauce to a boil.
4. Turn the heat down to medium-low, cover the pot, and simmer for 15 minutes, stirring occasionally.
5. Uncover the pot and simmer, stirring occasionally, for 15 minutes more.
6. While the sauce is simmering, cook the spaghetti until al dente according to the package instructions, with no salt added to the cooking water. Drain.
7. To serve, portion the spaghetti into six shallow bowls and spoon the sauce over the top, dividing it equally. Store leftovers in an airtight container in the refrigerator for 3 to 4 days.

SUBSTITUTION TIP: For fewer calories and carbs, swap the whole-wheat spaghetti for zucchini noodles.

PER SERVING: Calories: 408; Total Fat: 13g; Saturated Fat: 4g; Cholesterol: 49mg; Sodium: 70mg; Potassium: 676mg; Carbohydrates: 51g; Fiber: 8g; Sugars: 5g; Protein: 25g

Grilled Skirt Steak with Salsa Verde

Serves 4 / Prep time: 20 minutes / Cook time: 5 minutes, plus 5 minutes resting

Skirt steak is best served sliced across the grain to ensure tenderness. The lemon in the marinade tenderizes the steak by loosening the strands of muscle, all while adding fresh flavor, which is enhanced by the salsa verde.

FOR THE STEAK

1 (1½-pound) skirt steak
½ teaspoon freshly ground black pepper
¼ cup olive oil

Grated zest of 1 lemon
2 garlic cloves, minced

FOR THE SALSA VERDE

1 cup minced soft fresh herbs, such as
   mint, tarragon, or basil
1 cup minced fresh flat-leaf parsley
¼ cup olive oil

2 avocados, pitted and cut into
   ¼-inch dice
1 cup low-fat plain Greek yogurt

TO MAKE THE STEAK

1. Heat a grill to medium-high or heat a grill pan over medium-high heat.
2. In a large zip-top bag, sprinkle the steak with pepper. Add the oil, lemon zest, and garlic and stir to combine. Seal and let marinate for 20 minutes.
3. Grill the steak until charred, 2 to 3 minutes per side for medium-rare. Allow the beef to rest for 3 to 5 minutes before slicing.

TO MAKE SALSA VERDE

4. Meanwhile, in a medium bowl, toss the herbs, parsley, and oil. Stir in the avocado. Stir in the yogurt, ¼ cup at a time, until the salsa reaches a consistency you like.
5. Serve the steak with the salsa. Store leftovers in airtight containers, with the steak and salsa verde separately, in the refrigerator for 3 to 4 days.

PER SERVING: Calories: 730; Total Fat: 57g; Saturated Fat: 12g; Cholesterol: 119mg; Sodium: 151mg; Potassium: 1,312mg; Carbohydrates: 15g; Fiber: 7g; Sugars: 5g; Protein: 42g

Stuffed Flank Steak

Serves 6 / Prep time: 10 minutes / Cook time: 4 to 6 hours

You may not have cooked steak in the slow cooker before, but I guarantee it will be one of your new favorite meal preparations. Stuffed with savory aromatics, bright vegetables, and hearty nuts, this flank steak has every texture and flavor in one bite that you could desire. Serve with Peachy Tomato Salad (page 50) for a delicious pairing.

2 pounds flank steak
Freshly ground black pepper
1 tablespoon olive oil
¼ cup diced white onion
1 garlic clove, minced
2 cups chopped baby spinach

½ cup chopped dried tomatoes
½ cup diced roasted red peppers
½ cup raw unsalted almonds, toasted
  and chopped
½ cup low-sodium chicken broth

1. Lay the flank steak out on a cutting board and generously season with black pepper.
2. In a medium saucepan, heat the oil over medium heat. Add the onion and garlic. Cook, stirring frequently, for 5 minutes, or until onion is tender and translucent.
3. Add the spinach, tomatoes, roasted peppers, and almonds, and cook an additional 3 minutes, or until the spinach wilts slightly.
4. Let the tomato-spinach mixture cool to room temperature.
5. Spread the tomato-spinach mixture evenly over the flank steak. Roll the flank steak up slowly and tie it securely with kitchen twine on both ends and in the middle.
6. In the same pan, brown the flank steak for 5 minutes, turning it carefully to brown all sides.
7. Transfer the flank steak to a slow cooker. Add the broth to the bottom of the cooker and cover. Cook on low for 4 to 6 hours.
8. Cut the steak into rounds, discarding the twine, and serve. Store leftovers in an airtight container in the refrigerator for 3 to 4 days.

PER SERVING: Calories: 359; Total Fat: 21g; Saturated Fat: 6g; Cholesterol: 103mg; Sodium: 102mg; Potassium: 821mg; Carbohydrates: 7g; Fiber: 2g; Sugars: 3g; Protein: 35g

Spice-Rubbed Flank Steak with Tomato Jam

Serves 8 / Prep time: 10 minutes / Cook time: 25 minutes, plus 5 minutes resting

There is nothing like a hearty cut of meat at the center of your table, and you may be pleasantly surprised that you can still enjoy steak on the DASH diet. Lean cuts of animal protein are allowed on the diet, up to 6 ounces per day.

FOR THE TOMATO JAM

6 tomatoes (about 4 pounds), halved crosswise and cored

¼ cup sugar

⅓ cup grated white onion

3 garlic cloves, minced

2 jalapeños, seeded and minced

¼ cup chopped fresh cilantro

3 tablespoons freshly squeezed lime juice

FOR THE STEAK

2 teaspoons ground coriander

1 teaspoon ground cumin

1 teaspoon paprika

1 teaspoon freshly ground black pepper

1 teaspoon garlic powder

½ teaspoon ground cayenne pepper

2 pounds flank steak, fat trimmed

TO MAKE THE TOMATO JAM

1. Mince the tomatoes and place them with their juices in a medium saucepan. Add the sugar, onion, garlic, and jalapeños and bring to a boil over medium-high heat. Reduce the heat to medium-low and simmer, stirring occasionally, for about 20 minutes, until the mixture is reduced to about 2 cups. Remove from the heat and let cool.

TO MAKE THE STEAK

2. Heat a grill to high or heat a grill pan over high heat.
3. In a small bowl, combine the coriander, cumin, paprika, pepper, garlic powder, and cayenne. Rub the spice mixture all over the steak on both sides.

4. Place the steak on the grill and cook for about 3 minutes per side for medium-rare (4 or 5 minutes for more well-done). Remove from the heat and let rest for 5 minutes before slicing.
5. Stir the cilantro and lime juice into the jam right before serving with the steak.
6. To serve, slice the steak diagonally across the grain into ¼-inch-thick slices. Serve the sliced steak immediately, garnished with a dollop of the jam. Store leftover steak in an airtight container in the refrigerator for 3 to 4 days.

PREP TIP: The jam can be made ahead and stored in the refrigerator for up to a week. Bring it to room temperature before serving.

PER SERVING: Calories: 237; Total Fat: 10g; Saturated Fat: 4g; Cholesterol: 77mg; Sodium: 68mg; Potassium: 640mg; Carbohydrates: 12g; Fiber: 2g; Sugars: 9g; Protein: 25g

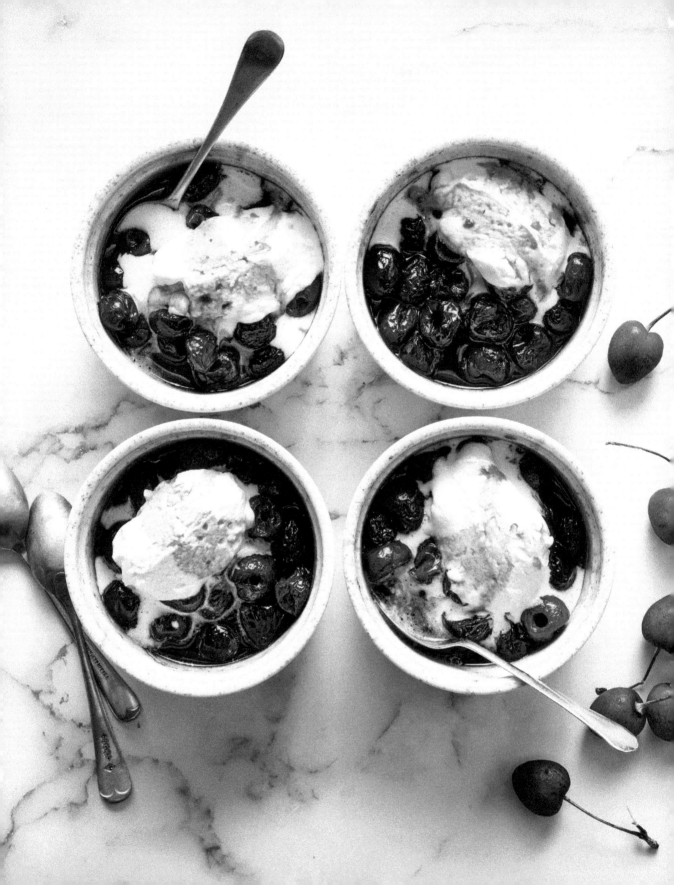

CHAPTER SEVEN

Staples, Snacks, and Sweets

Spiced Edamame

Serves 4 / Prep time: 5 minutes / Cook time: 15 minutes

Edamame is the immature soybean in the pod, and it is featured in the cuisines of Japan, China, and Hawaii. You can cook and season the pods for snacking, as we do here, or cook the shelled soybeans to use in salads and side dishes. To eat them from the pod, simply bite down on one end and pull the pod out between your clenched teeth. The beans pop out into your mouth along with the gentle flavors from the cooking broth.

2 tablespoons low-sodium soy sauce
2 tablespoons unseasoned rice vinegar
1 tablespoon brown sugar
3 garlic cloves, coarsely chopped
1 (10- to 14-ounce) package frozen
   edamame, thawed

1 tablespoon chili powder
1 teaspoon red pepper flakes
½ teaspoon dried oregano

1. Fill a medium pot half full of water and bring to a boil over medium-high heat. Add the soy sauce, rice vinegar, brown sugar, and garlic and stir well.
2. Add the edamame and boil for 6 to 8 minutes, until firm-tender. Drain well.
3. Transfer the edamame to a medium bowl and sprinkle with the chili powder, red pepper flakes, and oregano. Toss well to coat the pods evenly with the spices.
4. Serve immediately. Store leftovers in an airtight container in the refrigerator for 3 to 4 days.

PER SERVING: Calories: 106; Total Fat: 4g; Saturated Fat: 0g; Cholesterol: 0mg; Sodium: 319mg; Potassium: 426mg; Carbohydrates: 12g; Fiber: 4g; Sugars: 5g; Protein: 8g

Sweet-Hot Maple Almonds

Serves 6 / Prep time: 5 minutes / Cook time: 25 minutes

Almonds are a perfect protein-rich snack food when you're hungry and need some quick, delicious energy. In this recipe, the renowned flavor combination of sweet-hot—accomplished here by combining soy sauce and maple syrup—bakes into the nuts and turns them a deep mahogany color. Swap almonds for your favorite nut of choice.

1 pound raw unsalted almonds

5 tablespoons maple syrup

2 tablespoons low-sodium soy sauce

1 teaspoon ground cayenne pepper

Nonstick cooking spray

1. Preheat the oven to 350°F.
2. Spread the almonds in a single layer on a rimmed baking sheet and bake for 6 to 7 minutes. Let the almonds cool slightly; keep the oven on.
3. In a large bowl, whisk together the maple syrup, soy sauce, and cayenne. Add the almonds to the bowl and stir well until thoroughly coated.
4. Lightly coat the baking sheet with cooking spray. Spread the almonds over the pan in a single layer and roast for 15 to 17 minutes, stirring every few minutes, until the nuts turn a deep brown.
5. Let the almonds cool to room temperature before serving or storing. Store leftovers in an airtight container at room temperature for 1 week.

PER SERVING: Calories: 486; Total Fat: 38g; Saturated Fat: 3g; Cholesterol: 0mg; Sodium: 173mg; Potassium: 612mg; Carbohydrates: 28g; Fiber: 10g; Sugars: 13g; Protein: 16g

5 INGREDIENTS OR FEWER

30 MINUTES OR LESS

DAIRY-FREE

VEGAN

Baked Chili-Lime Tortilla Chips

Serves 4 / Prep time: 5 minutes / Cook time: 25 minutes

Given a choice between French fries and tortilla chips, many Americans would be hard pressed to pick a favorite. Luckily, we can take deep-fried out of the equation to comply with DASH and create these delicious baked chips—full of flavor for snacking on by themselves or equally perfect for scooping up a dip or salsa. Serve with Chipotle Guacamole (page 143) for a delicious, healthy snack.

12 (6-inch) corn tortillas
3 tablespoons canola oil or other vegetable oil

1 tablespoon chili powder
1 tablespoon grated lime zest
1 teaspoon ground cayenne pepper

1. Preheat the oven to 350°F.
2. Cut each tortilla into six wedges using kitchen shears or a sharp knife.
3. In a medium bowl, whisk together the oil, chili powder, lime zest, and cayenne. Dip the tortilla wedges in the oil mixture and spread in a single layer on two baking sheets or shallow roasting pans.
4. Bake for 20 to 25 minutes, until the chips are browned and crunchy. Transfer to paper towels to drain and cool before serving. Store leftovers in an airtight container at room temperature for 2 to 3 days.

PER SERVING: Calories: 258; Total Fat: 13g; Saturated Fat: 1g; Cholesterol: 0mg; Sodium: 90mg; Potassium: 186mg; Carbohydrates: 34g; Fiber: 5g; Sugars: 1g; Protein: 4g

Oil and Vinegar Roasted Chickpeas

Serves 4 / Prep time: 5 minutes, plus overnight to soak / Cook time: 1 hour 15 minutes

GLUTEN-FREE

DAIRY-FREE

NUT-FREE

VEGAN

Give chickpeas a crunchy exterior, and they become extremely addictive. If you have a snacking habit, chickpeas are a protein- and fiber-rich option. A serving of chickpeas is half the daily fiber required for adults. Add in the copper, calcium, potassium, and iron (26 percent of your daily needs) and you can't afford not to eat these delicious legumes. Note that the dried chickpeas need to be soaked overnight, so be sure to plan ahead when making this recipe.

3 cups dried chickpeas, soaked in water overnight

4 cups white vinegar

2 tablespoons olive oil

1 teaspoon coarse sea salt (optional)

1 teaspoon ground cayenne pepper

1 teaspoon grated lemon zest

½ teaspoon paprika

1. Preheat the oven to 400°F.
2. Drain the chickpeas. In a large saucepan, bring the vinegar to a boil over medium-high heat. Add the chickpeas and return to a boil. Watch closely; as soon as the liquid begins to boil, remove the pan from the heat and let the chickpeas sit in the hot vinegar for 30 minutes.
3. Drain the chickpeas, discarding the liquid, and then dry completely on paper towels.
4. In a large bowl, whisk together the oil, salt (if using), cayenne, lemon zest, and paprika. Add the chickpeas to the oil mixture, toss well to coat, then spread in a single layer on a rimmed baking sheet or shallow roasting pan.
5. Roast for about 45 minutes, checking and stirring the chickpeas every few minutes starting at 30 minutes to keep them from burning. Let cool and serve. Store leftovers in a glass container or bowl at room temperature for 1 to 2 days.

PREP TIP: Make this recipe even easier by using canned no-salt-added chickpeas, drained and rinsed, if you don't have time to soak the chickpeas overnight.

PER SERVING: Calories: 623; Total Fat: 14g; Saturated Fat: 2g; Cholesterol: 0mg; Sodium: 37mg; Potassium: 1,093mg; Carbohydrates: 95g; Fiber: 19g; Sugars: 16g; Protein: 31g

ONE-POT

30 MINUTES OR LESS

DAIRY-FREE

GLUTEN-FREE

NUT-FREE

VEGETARIAN

Herbed Deviled Eggs

Serves 6 / Prep time: 20 minutes

Deviled eggs are a classic potluck and holiday favorite. Luckily for cooks, there are countless additions to deviled eggs that make them really sing. Experiment until you find your very favorite combination. Add a few tablespoons of finely chopped celery or red bell pepper, use a reduced-fat mayonnaise, or play with different herbs and spices.

12 large hard-boiled eggs
3 tablespoons real mayonnaise, or
   1 tablespoon olive oil
1 tablespoon yellow mustard
1 tablespoon finely minced onion

1 tablespoon finely chopped fresh dill
1 teaspoon unseasoned rice vinegar
Freshly ground black pepper
Paprika, for garnish

1. Peel the eggs carefully. Slice them in half lengthwise and scoop the yolks into a medium bowl. Set the egg whites aside.
2. To the egg yolks, add the mayonnaise, mustard, onion, dill, and vinegar and mix with a fork until smooth. Season with pepper and adjust the flavor as needed.
3. Using a tablespoon or melon baller, scoop a small round of the egg yolk mixture and press carefully into an egg white. Repeat until all the egg whites are filled. Arrange the eggs on a platter, sprinkle with paprika, and serve.

INGREDIENT TIP: Most grocery stores carry peeled hard-boiled eggs. For added flavor and to make this snack more filling, top with Chipotle Guacamole (page 143).

PER SERVING: Calories: 176; Total Fat: 13g; Saturated Fat: 4g; Cholesterol: 374mg; Sodium: 231mg; Potassium: 160mg; Carbohydrates: 2g; Fiber: 0g; Sugars: 0g; Protein: 13g

Chipotle Guacamole

Serves 4 / Prep time: 5 minutes

Avocados are full of healthy fats that help prevent cardiovascular disease and diabetes while supporting weight maintenance and nutrient absorption. Serve with Baked Chili-Lime Tortilla Chips (page 140) for a healthy and delicious snack or party dish.

1 avocado

1 tomato, seeded and diced

1½ tablespoons finely diced red onion

1 tablespoon freshly squeezed lime juice

1 tablespoon minced fresh cilantro

⅛ to ¼ teaspoon ground chipotle

1. Halve the avocado, remove the pit, and use a large spoon to scoop out the flesh into a medium bowl. Mash the avocado with a fork, leaving it a bit lumpy.
2. Add the tomato, onion, lime juice, cilantro, and chipotle and stir to mix well.
3. Serve immediately. Store leftovers in an airtight container in the refrigerator for 1 to 2 days.

PER SERVING: Calories: 88; Total Fat: 7g; Saturated Fat: 1g; Cholesterol: 0mg; Sodium: 5mg; Potassium: 328mg; Carbohydrates: 6g; Fiber: 4g; Sugars: 1g; Protein: 1g

ONE-POT

30 MINUTES OR LESS

DAIRY-FREE

GLUTEN-FREE

NUT-FREE

VEGAN

ONE-POT

30 MINUTES OR LESS

DAIRY-FREE

GLUTEN-FREE

NUT-FREE

VEGAN

Roasted Red Pepper Hummus

Serves 6 / Prep time: 5 minutes

Store-bought hummus, while full of protein, fiber, vitamins, and minerals, usually contains high amounts of sodium. This homemade version is quick to make and relies on roasted peppers and spices, not salt, for flavor. Serve this tasty dip with crudités or whole-wheat pita triangles for a healthy snack or appetizer.

1 (15-ounce) can no-salt-added chickpeas, drained and rinsed
½ cup jarred roasted red bell peppers, drained
1 garlic clove, peeled

¼ cup freshly squeezed lemon juice
2 tablespoons tahini
1 tablespoon olive oil
¼ teaspoon ground cumin
⅛ teaspoon ground cayenne pepper

1. In a food processor, combine the chickpeas, red peppers, and garlic and process until smooth.
2. Add the lemon juice, tahini, oil, cumin, and cayenne, and process to blend well. If the mixture is too thick, add water, 1 tablespoon at a time, until it reaches the desired consistency.
3. Serve immediately or store in an airtight container in the refrigerator for up to 3 days.

PER SERVING: Calories: 123; Total Fat: 6g; Saturated Fat: 1g; Cholesterol: 0mg; Sodium: 9mg; Potassium: 173mg; Carbohydrates: 14g; Fiber: 4g; Sugars: 3g; Protein: 5g

Spicy Nutty Granola

Serves 6 / Prep time: 10 minutes / Cook time: 30 minutes

Granola makes an excellent snack, breakfast topping, and pairing with yogurt, cheese, or fruit. Double this recipe and store the leftovers in the refrigerator, where it will keep for about a week and a half. If you don't have time to squeeze your own orange juice, use store-bought juice with the pulp.

¼ cup freshly squeezed orange juice
¼ cup honey
2 tablespoons canola oil
1 cup old-fashioned oats
1 cup raw unsalted almonds
1 cup raw unsalted walnuts

¼ cup sesame seeds
¼ cup flaxseeds
1 tablespoon grated orange zest
1 teaspoon ground cinnamon
½ teaspoon ground nutmeg
½ teaspoon ground ginger

1. Preheat the oven to 350°F.
2. In a small bowl, mix the orange juice, honey, and oil together and set aside.
3. In a large bowl, mix the oats, almonds, walnuts, sesame seeds, flaxseeds, orange zest, cinnamon, nutmeg, and ginger until well combined. Drizzle the oil mixture over the dry ingredients and stir until evenly coated.
4. Pack the mixture tightly into a 9-by-13-inch glass baking dish and bake for 30 minutes, until golden brown.
5. Let cool completely, then break into chunks and store in an airtight container at room temperature for up to 1 week.

PER SERVING: Calories: 466; Total fat: 35g; Saturated fat: 3g; Cholesterol: 0mg; Sodium: 7mg; Potassium: 409mg; Carbohydrates: 33g; Fiber: 9g; Sugars: 14g; Protein: 12g

ONE-POT

5 INGREDIENTS OR FEWER

30 MINUTES OR LESS

GLUTEN-FREE

NUT-FREE

VEGETARIAN

Pumpkin Vanilla Pudding

Serves 6 / Prep time: 10 minutes

This decadent dessert will make you think you're cheating on the DASH diet when, in fact, you're not. Sure to please your sweet tooth, this pudding delivers fiber, antioxidants, and beta carotene. This smooth, luscious dessert is equally tasty served warm or cold.

1½ cups low-fat vanilla yogurt
1 (20-ounce) can pure pumpkin puree
½ teaspoon ground nutmeg

½ teaspoon ground cinnamon
1 vanilla bean, halved lengthwise

1. In a medium bowl, combine the yogurt, pumpkin puree, nutmeg, and cinnamon. Scrape the vanilla seeds out of the pod into the bowl; discard the pod.
2. Mix well until all ingredients are combined. Chill until ready to serve. Store leftovers in an airtight container in the refrigerator for 3 to 4 days.

SUBSTITUTION TIP: If you don't have or can't find a vanilla bean, substitute 1 teaspoon vanilla extract.

PER SERVING: Calories: 72; Total Fat: 1g; Saturated Fat: 1g; Cholesterol: 0mg; Sodium: 48mg; Potassium: 340mg; Carbohydrates: 12g; Fiber: 3g; Sugars: 7g; Protein: 4g

Strawberry-Banana Frozen Yogurt

Serves 16 / Prep time: 10 minutes, plus 4 hours to chill

Nonfat and low-fat plain yogurt are go-to ingredients in the DASH diet, especially Greek yogurt. Even in its nonfat form, Greek yogurt is thick and rich—plus, it has more protein and about 40 percent less sodium than regular yogurt. Swap out the strawberries for raspberries, blueberries, mango, or another fruit of your choice.

3 cups low-fat plain Greek yogurt

3 ripe bananas

2 cups frozen strawberries, thawed, with
   their juice

1 cup crushed pineapple, canned
   in juice

1. Line 16 muffin cups with the paper liners.
2. Combine the yogurt, bananas, strawberries, and pineapple in a blender or food processor. Blend until smooth.
3. Spoon the yogurt mixture into the prepared muffin cups and freeze until firm, about 4 hours.
4. To serve, peel off the paper and let the frozen yogurt stand for 10 minutes. To save the frozen yogurt for later, take the cups out of the muffin tin and put them back in the freezer in a sealed container or a heavy plastic zip-top bag. Store frozen for up to 1 month.

PER SERVING: Calories: 68; Total Fat: 1g; Saturated Fat: 0g; Cholesterol: 3mg; Sodium: 33mg; Potassium: 247mg; Carbohydrates: 13g; Fiber: 1g; Sugars: 9g; Protein: 3g

ONE-POT

5 INGREDIENTS OR FEWER

30 MINUTES OR LESS

GLUTEN-FREE

DAIRY-FREE

VEGETARIAN

Roasted Plums with Greek Yogurt

Serves 4 / Prep time: 5 minutes / Cook time: 15 minutes

Roasting fruit intensifies its sweetness and brings out a caramelized flavor. These roasted plums are paired with a dollop of yogurt and a sprinkling of hazelnuts for a midday snack or healthful dessert.

6 plums, halved and pitted
Nonstick cooking spray
½ cup low-fat plain Greek yogurt

2 tablespoons chopped hazelnuts, toasted
2 teaspoons honey

1. Preheat the oven to 375°F. Line a baking sheet with parchment paper.
2. Arrange the plums cut-side up on the baking sheet and spray with cooking spray. Bake the plums until they begin to soften and brown a bit, about 15 minutes.
3. Divide the plums evenly among four serving bowls and top each with a dollop of yogurt, a sprinkle of nuts, and a drizzle of honey. Serve immediately. Store leftovers in an airtight container in the refrigerator for 2 to 3 days.

SUBSTITUTION TIP: In the summertime, opt for fresh ripe peaches instead of plums to mix this recipe up.

PER SERVING: Calories: 99; Total Fat: 3g; Saturated Fat: 0g; Cholesterol: 2mg; Sodium: 22mg; Potassium: 253mg; Carbohydrates: 17g; Fiber: 2g; Sugars: 15g; Protein: 3g

Figs Baked with Goat Cheese and Honey

Serves 4 / Prep time: 10 minutes / Cook time: 10 minutes

What could be a better dessert than one that benefits your health? Figs help the heart with lots of potassium and the waistline with lots of fiber. Walnuts are full of omega-3 fatty acids, good for the human heart and brain. Swap out the goat cheese for ricotta, if you prefer.

4 large fresh figs, halved
4 ounces goat cheese
2 tablespoons honey

Freshly ground black pepper
¼ cup raw unsalted walnut pieces

1. Preheat the oven to 350°F.
2. Arrange the figs cut-side up on a rimmed baking sheet or in a shallow roasting pan.
3. Spoon ½ tablespoon of the goat cheese on each fig half, then drizzle with ¼ tablespoon of the honey. Bake for 5 to 8 minutes, just until the cheese has softened.
4. Arrange two fig halves on each dessert plate, topping them with another drizzle of honey, if desired. Season the figs lightly with pepper and scatter with walnuts. Serve immediately.

PER SERVING: Calories: 202; Total Fat: 11g; Saturated Fat: 5g; Cholesterol: 13mg; Sodium: 131mg; Potassium: 194mg; Carbohydrates: 22g; Fiber: 2g; Sugars: 19g; Protein: 7g

ONE-POT

5 INGREDIENTS OR FEWER

30 MINUTES OR LESS

GLUTEN-FREE

VEGETARIAN

Port-Roasted Red Cherries with Vanilla Whipped "Cream"

Serve 4 / Prep time: 15 minutes / Cook time: 15 minutes

Cherries are an antioxidant-rich fruit choice that are delicious fresh or baked. The deep flavor pairs well with the port and is lifted with the light, airy whipped topping, which you'd never guess is low-fat!

FOR THE CHERRIES

Nonstick cooking spray
1 pound red cherries, pitted

4 tablespoons ruby port

FOR THE WHIPPED TOPPING

1 large egg white
2 tablespoons granulated sugar
¼ teaspoon cream of tartar

¼ cup low-fat evaporated milk, chilled
½ teaspoon vanilla extract

TO MAKE THE CHERRIES

1. Preheat the oven to 450°F. Spray four 8-ounce ramekins with cooking spray and place them on a rimmed baking sheet.
2. Divide the cherries evenly among the prepared ramekins. Bake until the cherries soften and become juicy, about 10 minutes. Remove the ramekins from the oven and drizzle 1 tablespoon of the port into each. Stir to coat the cherries. Return the pan to the oven and bake until the liquid begins to bubble and thicken, about 5 minutes.

TO MAKE THE WHIPPED TOPPING

3. While the cherries are roasting, combine the egg white and sugar in the top of a double boiler over simmering water and heat gently, whisking constantly, until the mixture is warm and the sugar is completely dissolved. Test this by dipping your fingers into the mixture; if the mixture feels smooth, not grainy, it is ready.

4. Transfer the egg white mixture to a large bowl. Add the cream of tartar and, using an electric mixer, beat on medium-high speed for about 3 minutes, until stiff peaks form. Whisk in the evaporated milk and vanilla. Beat until the mixture holds soft peaks, about 3 minutes.
5. Serve the cherries warm, topped with a dollop of the whipped topping.

PER SERVING: Calories: 126; Total Fat: 1g; Saturated Fat: 0g; Cholesterol: 1mg; Sodium: 36mg; Potassium: 308mg; Carbohydrates: 24g; Fiber: 2g; Sugars: 19g; Protein: 3g

Peach-Blueberry Crisp with Coconut Topping

Serves 4 / Prep time: 5 minutes / Cook time: 10 minutes

Fruit crisps are a dessert that can be made year-round with apples but are made even more delicious when stone fruits and berries are at their peak. In the fall, you might substitute apples or pears and cranberries. Cooking the crisp in individual ramekins ensures that both portion control and cleanup are a snap. Be sure to use ramekins that are microwave- and oven-safe.

FOR THE FILLING

Nonstick cooking spray
2 cups sliced fresh peaches
1 cup fresh blueberries

2 tablespoons all-purpose flour
2 tablespoons freshly squeezed
   lemon juice

FOR THE TOPPING

¾ cup old-fashioned oats
¼ cup all-purpose flour
¼ cup packed brown sugar

3 tablespoons unsweetened
   coconut flakes
2 tablespoons tub margarine

TO MAKE THE FILLING

1. Spray four 8-ounce ramekins lightly with cooking spray.
2. In a large bowl, toss the peaches and blueberries. Add the flour and lemon juice and toss to combine. Spoon the mixture equally among the prepared ramekins. Cover the ramekins tightly with plastic wrap and make a few small holes in each. Cook on high in the microwave for 5 to 7 minutes, until the filling is hot and bubbling.

TO MAKE THE TOPPING

3. While the filling is cooking, preheat the broiler to high.
4. In a food processor, combine the oats, flour, brown sugar, coconut flakes, and margarine. Pulse until the mixture is well combined.
5. Remove the ramekins from the microwave, remove and discard the plastic wrap, and place the ramekins on a baking sheet. Spoon the topping mixture over the fruit in the ramekins, making sure to cover the fruit completely.
6. Place the baking sheet with the filled ramekins under the broiler and broil for 2 to 3 minutes, until the topping is nicely browned.
7. Serve warm. Store leftovers in an airtight container in the refrigerator for 3 to 4 days.

PER SERVING: Calories: 271; Total Fat: 9g; Saturated Fat: 2g; Cholesterol: 0mg; Sodium: 8mg; Potassium: 284mg; Carbohydrates: 47g; Fiber: 4g; Sugars: 24g; Protein: 4g

No-Bake Chocolate-Glazed Coconut Bars

Makes 8 bars / Prep time: 25 minutes / Cook time: 5 minutes

These snack or dessert bars seem sinful, when they are actually incredibly heart-healthy. They contain healthy fat from the coconut as well as antioxidants from the dark chocolate. Talk about healthy food turned candy treat!

FOR THE BARS

1½ cups unsweetened shredded coconut
2 tablespoons sugar
2 tablespoons coconut cream

2 tablespoons olive oil
½ teaspoon vanilla extract

FOR THE CHOCOLATE GLAZE

3 tablespoons mini dark chocolate chips

1½ teaspoons tub margarine

TO MAKE THE BARS

1. In a medium bowl, stir together the coconut, sugar, coconut cream, oil, and vanilla until well combined. Press the mixture into an 8-inch square baking pan.
2. Chill in the freezer for 15 minutes, until firm.

TO MAKE THE CHOCOLATE GLAZE

3. Meanwhile, line a baking sheet with parchment paper.
4. In a microwave-safe glass measuring cup with a spout or a small microwave-safe bowl, combine the chocolate chips and margarine. Heat in the microwave in 30-second increments until the chocolate chips are halfway melted. Stir to melt them completely and combine the mixture well.

5. Remove the pan from the freezer and cut the mixture into eight bars. Place the bars on the prepared baking sheet and drizzle the chocolate glaze over the top. Place the baking sheet in the freezer for about 5 minutes, until the chocolate has set. Serve immediately or store in an airtight container in the refrigerator for up to 3 weeks.

PER SERVING (1 BAR): Calories: 137; Total Fat: 12g; Saturated Fat: 7g; Cholesterol: 0mg; Sodium: 4mg; Potassium: 93mg; Carbohydrates: 7g; Fiber: 2g; Sugars: 5g; Protein: 1g

Fruit and Chocolate-Studded Oatmeal Cookies

Makes 40 cookies / Prep time: 10 minutes / Cook time: 15 minutes

Yogurt and plant oils add excellent moisture and flavor to cookies in place of butter. Dried fruit and dark chocolate chips make these cookies seem like an indulgence, but they're actually cholesterol-free and full of healthful nutrients. Like many other sweets, these cookies do contain added sugar, so try to limit intake to a weekly treat.

1⅓ cups old-fashioned or
   quick-cooking oats
1 cup whole-wheat flour
¼ cup packed brown sugar
1 teaspoon baking powder
1 teaspoon ground cinnamon
¼ teaspoon ground mace

⅓ cup low-fat plain yogurt
1 large egg
2 tablespoons canola oil
1 teaspoon vanilla extract
½ cup chopped mixed dried fruit
½ cup dark chocolate chips

1. Preheat the oven to 350°F. Line two baking sheets with silicone baking mats or parchment paper.
2. In a medium bowl, combine the oats, flour, brown sugar, baking powder, cinnamon, and mace and mix well.
3. In a large bowl, mix the yogurt, egg, oil, and vanilla. Add the flour mixture to the yogurt mixture. Using a spatula, mix until just combined. Stir in the dried fruit and chocolate chips.
4. Using a tablespoon, drop heaping tablespoons of the dough onto the prepared baking sheets, spacing them about 2 inches apart.
5. Bake for 10 to 12 minutes, until lightly browned. Remove from the oven and let cool on a wire rack. Store in an airtight container at room temperature for up to 1 week.

INGREDIENT TIP: Use gluten-free oats and gluten-free flour to make these cookies gluten-free. (Make sure the baking powder you use is also naturally gluten-free.)

PER SERVING (2 COOKIES): Calories: 104; Total Fat: 4g; Saturated Fat: 1g; Cholesterol: 10mg; Sodium: 9mg; Potassium: 138mg; Carbohydrates: 16g; Fiber: 2g; Sugars: 6g; Protein: 2g

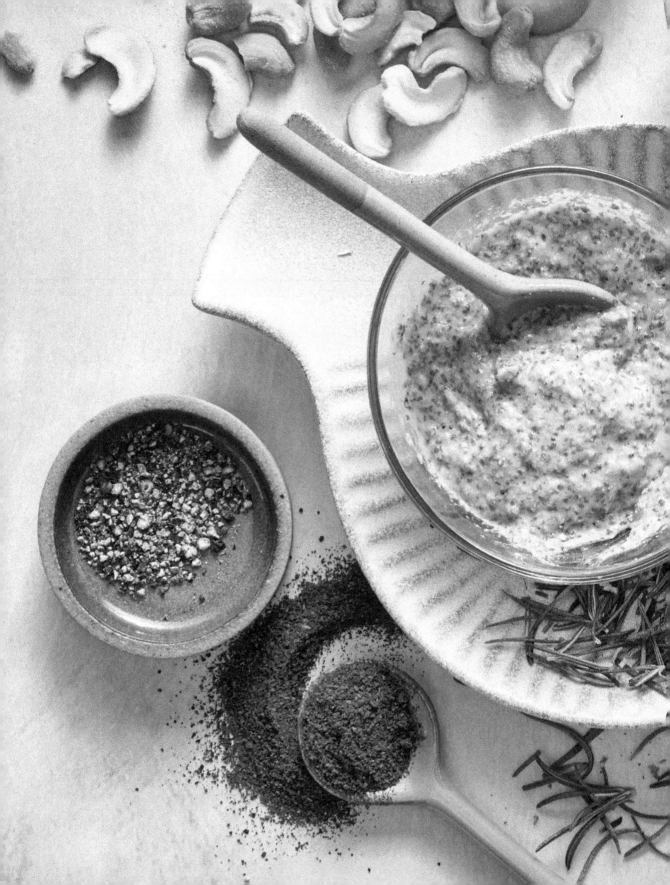

Measurement Conversions

	US Standard	US Standard (ounces)	Metric (approximate)
VOLUME EQUIVALENTS (LIQUID)	2 tablespoons	1 fl. oz.	30 mL
	¼ cup	2 fl. oz.	60 mL
	½ cup	4 fl. oz.	120 mL
	1 cup	8 fl. oz.	240 mL
	1½ cups	12 fl. oz.	355 mL
	2 cups or 1 pint	16 fl. oz.	475 mL
	4 cups or 1 quart	32 fl. oz.	1 L
	1 gallon	128 fl. oz.	4 L
VOLUME EQUIVALENTS (DRY)	⅛ teaspoon		0.5 mL
	¼ teaspoon		1 mL
	½ teaspoon		2 mL
	¾ teaspoon		4 mL
	1 teaspoon		5 mL
	1 tablespoon		15 mL
	¼ cup		59 mL
	⅓ cup		79 mL
	½ cup		118 mL
	⅔ cup		156 mL
	¾ cup		177 mL
	1 cup		235 mL
	2 cups or 1 pint		475 mL
	3 cups		700 mL
	4 cups or 1 quart		1 L
	½ gallon		2 L
	1 gallon		4 L
WEIGHT EQUIVALENTS	½ ounce		15 g
	1 ounce		30 g
	2 ounces		60 g
	4 ounces		115 g
	8 ounces		225 g
	12 ounces		340 g
	16 ounces or 1 pound		455 g

	Fahrenheit (F)	Celsius (C) (approximate)
OVEN TEMPERATURES	250°F	120°C
	300°F	150°C
	325°F	180°C
	375°F	190°C
	400°F	200°C
	425°F	220°C
	450°F	230°C

Resources

The Academy of Nutrition and Dietetics, *eatright.org*

National Heart, Lung and Institute, *nhlbi.nih.gov/health-topics/dash-eating-plan*

American Heart Association, *heart.org/en/healthy-living/healthy-eating/eat-smart /nutrition-basics/aha-diet-and-lifestyle-recommendations*

DASH for Health, *dashforhealth.com*

DASH Diet support groups, *dashdiet.org/dash-support-group.html*

References

AMERICAN HEART ASSOCIATION. "Changes You Can Make to Manage High Blood Pressure." Accessed February 24, 2021. heart.org/en /health-topics/high-blood-pressure/changes-you-can-make-to -manage-high-blood-pressure/getting-active-to-control-high -blood-pressure.

AMERICAN HEART ASSOCIATION. "Understanding Blood Pressure Readings." Accessed February 24, 2021. heart.org/en/health -topics/high-blood-pressure/understanding-blood-pressure -readings.

CENTERS FOR DISEASE CONTROL AND PREVENTION. "About High Blood Pressure." Accessed February 24, 2021. CDC.gov/bloodpressure /about.htm.

CENTERS FOR DISEASE CONTROL AND PREVENTION. "High Blood Pressure Facts." Accessed February 24, 2021. CDC.gov/bloodpressure /facts.htm.

EVERETT, BETHANY AND ANNA ZAJACOVA. "Gender Differences in Hypertension and Hypertension Awareness among Young Adults."

Biodemography and Social Biology 61, no. 1 (2015): 1–17. Accessed February 24, 2021. ncbi.nlm.nih.gov/pmc/articles/PMC4896734/. DOI: 10.1080/19485565.2014.929488.

GUNNARS, KRIS. "12 Proven Health Benefits of Avocados." *Healthline*. Published June 29, 2018. Accessed February 26, 2021. Healthline.com/nutrition/12-proven-benefits-of-avocado.

HABIB, LISA. "Low-Fat Dairy Lowers Blood Pressure." Published June 26, 2006. Accessed February 24, 2021. WebMD.com/hypertension-high -blood-pressure/news/20060626/low-fat-dairy-lowers-blood -pressure.

JOHNS HOPKINS MEDICINE. "Exercise and the Heart." Accessed February 24, 2021. HopkinsMedicine.org/health/wellness-and -prevention/exercise-and-the-heart.

KLEMM, SARAH. "DASH Eating Plan: Reducing Blood Pressure through Diet and Lifestyle." *Academy of Nutrition and Dietetics.* Published February 11, 2021. Accessed February 24, 2021. eatright.org/health /wellness/heart-and-cardiovascular-health/dash-diet-reducing -hypertension-through-diet-and-lifestyle.

MARCIN, JUDITH. "Everything You Need to Know about High Blood Pressure." *Healthline.* Accessed February 24, 2021. healthline.com /health/high-blood-pressure-hypertension#overview.

MAYO CLINIC. "Dash Diet." Accessed February 24, 2021. MayoClinic.org /healthy-lifestyle/nutrition-and-healthy-eating/in-depth/dash-diet /art-20050989.

MAYO CLINIC. "High Blood Pressure." Accessed February 24, 2021. MayoClinic.org/diseases-conditions/high-blood-pressure /symptoms-causes/syc-20373410.

MAYO CLINIC. "High Blood Pressure." Accessed February 24, 2021. MayoClinic.org/diseases-conditions/high-blood-pressure /in-depth/high-blood-pressure/art-20045206.

MAYO CLINIC. "Nutrition and Healthy Eating." Accessed February 24, 2021. MayoClinic.org/healthy-lifestyle/nutrition-and-healthy-eating/in-depth/dash-diet/art-20048456.

MAYO CLINIC. "Whole Grain Foods." Accessed February 24, 2021. MayoClinic.org/diseases-conditions/high-blood-pressure/expert-answers/whole-grain-foods/faq-20058417.

SAEE, ANUM, DAVE L. DIXON, AND EUGENE YANG. "Racial Disparities in Hypertension Prevalence and Management: A Crisis Control?" Published April 6, 2020. Accessed February 24, 2021. Acc.org/latest-in-cardiology/articles/2020/04/06/08/53/racial-disparities-in-hypertension-prevalence-and-management.

U.S. DEPARTMENT OF HEALTH & HUMAN SERVICES. "DASH Eating Plan." Accessed February 24, 2021. nhlbi.nih.gov/health-topics/dash-eating-plan.

U.S. DEPARTMENT OF HEALTH & HUMAN SERVICES. "High Blood Pressure." Accessed February 24, 2021. nhlbi.nih.gov/health-topics/high-blood-pressure.

U.S. NATIONAL LIBRARY OF MEDICINE. "DASH Eating Plan." *MedlinePlus.* Accessed February 24, 2021. MedlinePlus.gov/dasheatingplan.html.

WEST, HELEN. "The Complete Beginner's Guide to the DASH Diet." *Healthline.* Published October 17, 2018. Accessed February 24, 2021. healthline.com/nutrition/dash-diet.

Index

Acknowledgments

The team at Callisto deserves so much credit for the publication of this book; it was a brilliant team effort, and I am so happy to be a part of bringing this book to readers.

About the Author

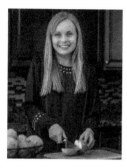

Amanda Foote, RD, is a registered dietitian, author, proud fire wife, and mother. It is her calling to ensure that food remains an enjoyable, nourishing part of the human experience. Amanda has worked as a registered dietitian for InnovAge and South Adams County Fire Department, as well as in private practice. Amanda has a bachelor's degree in dietetics from the University of Northern Colorado and a bachelor's degree in applied psychology from Regis University.

Printed in the USA
CPSIA information can be obtained
at www.ICGtesting.com
CBHW080818300124
3674CB00011B/2

9 781648 763267